DBT NEXT STEPS SKILLS HANDOUTS

Also Available

DBT Next Steps Skills Handouts

Building a Life Worth Living

Katherine Anne Comtois
Adam Carmel
Marsha M. Linehan

gp

THE GUILFORD PRESS
New York   London

The authors have checked with sources believed to be reliable in their efforts to provide information
that is complete and generally in accord with the standards of practice that are accepted at the time of
publication. However, in view of the possibility of human error or changes in behavioral, mental health,
or medical sciences, neither the authors, nor the editor and publisher, nor any other party who has been
involved in the preparation or publication of this work warrants that the information contained herein
is in every respect accurate or complete, and they are not responsible for any errors or omissions or the
results obtained from the use of such information. Readers are encouraged to confirm the information
contained in this book with other sources.

ISBN 978-1-4625-5816-2 (paperback) ISBN 978-1-4625-5817-9 (hardcover)

About the Authors

Katherine Anne Comtois, PhD, MPH, is Professor in the Department of Psychiatry and Behavioral Sciences and Adjunct Professor in the Department of Psychology at the University of Washington. She was a research therapist and co-investigator with Marsha Linehan on her clinical trials from 1994 to 2006 and Director of the DBT program at Harborview Mental Health and Addiction Services from 1996 to 2019. She now leads the DBT clinic and training program at the University of Washington Medical Center Outpatient Psychiatry Clinic. Dr. Comtois provides training and consultation on DBT Next Steps and the DBT-ACES program through the University of Washington. In addition, Dr. Comtois provides training and consultation in standard DBT internationally as an independent contractor with Treatment Implementation Collaborative LLC.

Adam Carmel, PhD, is Clinical Professor in the Department of Psychiatry and Behavioral Sciences at the University of Washington. He is Codirector of the Annual Comprehensive DBT Training program in the Department of Psychiatry and Behavioral Sciences at the University of Washington. He was previously Director of the Massachusetts Mental Health Center's DBT program operated by the Massachusetts Department of Mental Health. Dr. Carmel was previously Clinical Assistant Professor in the Department of Psychology at the University of Washington, where he taught DBT in the Behavioral Research and Therapy Clinics under the direction of Marsha Linehan.

Marsha M. Linehan, PhD, ABPP, the developer of Dialectical Behavior Therapy (DBT), is Professor Emeritus of Psychology and Director Emeritus of the Behavioral Research and Therapy Clinics at the University of Washington. Before retiring in 2019, she devoted her career to developing and evaluating evidence-based treatments for populations with high suicide risk and multiple, severe mental disorders. Dr. Linehan is the 2025 recipient of the Lifetime Achievement Award from the American Foundation for Suicide Prevention. Her contributions to suicide research and clinical psychology research have also been recognized with the University of Louisville Grawemeyer Award for Psychology, the Career/Lifetime Achievement Award from the Association for Behavioral and Cognitive Therapies, the Gold Medal Award for Life Achievement in the Application of Psychology from the American Psychological Foundation, and the James McKeen Cattell Award from the Association for Psychological Science. In her honor, the American Association of Suicidology created the Marsha Linehan Award for Outstanding Research in the Treatment of Suicidal Behavior. Dr. Linehan was featured in *TIME Great Scientists: The Geniuses and Visionaries Who Transformed Our World*. She is founder of the Linehan Institute and is a Zen master.

Preface

Featuring over 48 handouts and assignments, this skills-training manual includes all of the fundamental skills of DBT Next Steps. These innovative skills offer a way to stretch across the divide for the client who successfully completed Standard DBT and hasn't achieved their life worth living ambitions to work, go to school, or be self-sufficient. In this manual, you will find useful and accessible content on DBT Next Steps skills training and overall structure and contingencies that are needed in order to make significant progress and gain momentum toward life worth living goals.

This manual includes all of the components of DBT Next Steps skills, including the handouts used for skills training and assignments used for skills practice. For DBT Next Steps skills, the word "assignments" is used instead of "homework" or "worksheets" because this word is more general to work, not just school, contexts. One goal of DBT Next Steps is for the client to practice professional behavior in treatment even when feeling emotionally vulnerable or annoyed, and definitely when they don't feel like it. Completing an "assignment" of skills practice is an opportunity to rehearse professional behavior during skills training—similar to how one would want to approach an assigned task in a work setting.

DBT Next Steps are the skills we developed for a treatment called DBT-ACES (Accepting the Challenges of Employment and Self-Sufficiency), a comprehensive program designed to help clients find and maintain living wage employment (see pp. 7–8 for more information). These skills were developed over a period of 20 years at the University of Washington and Harborview Mental Health and Addiction Services. While DBT Next Steps skills are an important part of DBT-ACES, they can also be practiced on their own or incorporated into DBT and other treatments.

These expanded skills modules focus on understanding principles of reinforcement, considering alternatives to perfectionism, establishing and re-evaluating relationships and community mapping, managing time effectively, succeeding in usual care after DBT, and utilizing advanced strategies to apply mindfulness techniques and to regulate emotions. Through this novel DBT Next Steps Skills-Training Curriculum, clients will create new capabilities to achieve their employment, relationship, and independence goals. Our companion guide, *DBT Next Steps Clinician's Manual,* includes detailed lesson plans for each of the DBT Next Steps skills as well as detailed information for leading DBT Next Steps groups and other strategies that can be incorporated into individual therapy or used comprehensively in a DBT-ACES program. Other essential DBT Next Steps materials are available free of charge at www.dbtnextsteps.com.

Acknowledgments

We would like to acknowledge the many partners who made this skills-training manual possible. We want to thank the Harborview DBT Program clinicians who spent hours with Kate developing and refining these handouts through their many iterations starting with Marty Hoiness, MD; then Kristina Campbell, LMHC; then Lynn Elwood, LMHC, and Cristina Mullen, LICSW; then Jenna Melman, LICSW, and Mike McDonell, PhD; and finally, Britt Alvy, LICSW. We want to acknowledge Harborview DBT clinicians Wayne Smith, PhD; JoAnn Marsden, BA RT; and Penni Brinkerhoff, LMHC; as well as Lynn McFarr, PhD, Lisa Bolden, PsyD, and others at the Harbor–UCLA DBT-ACES program; and Klaus and Stephanie Höeschel in the German DBT-ACES program who led DBT Next Steps groups during formative stages and provided key input. The National Institute of Mental Health and the Catherine Wilkins Foundation provided critical financial support allowing us to evaluate and improve the program. DBT Next Steps clients have tried our new skills, given positive and negative feedback, and ensured that these skills would be widely acceptable and useful. Finally, Adam and Kate would like to acknowledge Marsha Linehan's core work on which DBT Next Steps was built and our successful collaboration with her in bringing this program to be. Thank you, Marsha.

Contents

PART I

DBT NEXT STEPS OVERVIEW

Skills-Training Syllabus

General Format

(Times are approximate depending on size of class and amount of homework.)

5 minutes	Good News
30–50 minutes	Ambitions and Action Steps Check-In

    1. What ambition are you working toward?

    2. What Action Steps(s) did you work on last week?

    3. What Employment Step(s) are you working on? What is your deadline?

    4. What progress have you made on your Action Step?

    5. What is something effective that you did to reach your Action Step?

    6. What have you done to avoid working on your Action Step? How will you not do this again?

    7. What emotion did you observe?

    8. What are your Action and Employment Steps for next week?

10–15 minutes	Break
15–30 minutes	Review of Assignments
20–30 minutes	New Material

New Material Syllabus

Month

_____   Perfectionism versus Reinforcement

_____   Establishing and Re-Evaluating Relationships

_____   Time Management

_____   Managing Emotions Effectively

_____   Succeeding after DBT

_____   Applications of Mindfulness

If completing a second round of the skills:

_____   Perfectionism versus Reinforcement

_____   Establishing and Re-Evaluating Relationships

_____   Time Management

_____   Managing Emotions Effectively

_____   Succeeding after DBT

_____   Applications of Mindfulness

DBT Next Steps Skills Group Participation Guidelines

Good News

You are not required to have good news every week. At the same time, we encourage you to be mindful of what is *not* going wrong during the week and speak up about it.

Check-In

1. *Complete your check-in sheet BEFORE* group starts, including a first draft of your new Action and Employment Steps for next week (we may revise this during group). Consider your life ambition as a work in progress that evolves over time. See Appendix 3: Overview of the Role of the Life Ambition in DBT Next Steps.

2. Stay mindful. Don't check out during others' Check-Ins.

   a. When others have achieved their Action Step, reinforce them verbally or nonverbally in a way that works for them. (This takes practice, as some folks like a lot of attention and others don't. Learning to "read the room" is a great skill.)

   b. When others can't figure out how to prevent avoidance or what their new Action Step should be, participate in the discussion with questions and ideas. (Again, read their nonverbals to see if you are helping or whether they are working it out for themselves or listening to someone else's idea.)

3. *If you miss group, don't stagnate.* Do a Check-In on your own and come up with a new Action and Employment Step to do and review the next week in class.

Assignments

- Complete assignments *BEFORE* you come to group and be sure to *write them down*. Make corrections based on feedback so your skills book has correct examples you can use to remember these skills down the road.

- We may not have a lot of time for each person, so think *BEFORE* group if there are key observations you want to make or questions you want to ask.

- If you miss a group, the assignment is on the first page of each module. Please review the material you missed and prepare the assignment, so you are at the same place as everyone else the following week.

(continued)

- If you did not review an assignment in group (because you missed or did not have your assignment done), show the co-leader it is done *outside of class or during a break* ASAP. If you have questions about past assignments, ask them then.
- Do not let late assignments linger. The material moves quickly, so you need to stay with the group.
- If you missed an assignment, you are expected to complete it ASAP. If you are four or more assignments behind, you will be on suspension until you've got less than four due.
- We do not track which assignments you have completed, only the number you are behind. We consider an assignment completed if you have written it out. So, if you don't remember what assignments are due, check your skills book and see what you haven't completed.
- Remember, the group leaders are like your supervisors or college professors. Don't make us chase you for assignments. Be proactive in coming to us with them completed. (Ask your individual therapist for help, if needed.)

New Material

Please *take written notes* when new material is presented: Our goal is for your skills book to be an effective reference down the road. Ask questions or share your observations. Teaching is designed as a seminar with lots of discussion.

Practice Professional Behavior in DBT Next Steps

One goal of DBT Next Steps is to not only find and keep a job, but also to be the employee given *raises, promotions*, and *great references*. This requires professional behavior—even when feeling vulnerable or annoyed and definitely when you don't feel like it.

Unprofessional behavior tends to be remembered a long time, even in the face of nothing but professional behavior since. The best way to prevent an unprofessional moment from being remembered is to have it be so unusual that it is dismissed as irrelevant. That means laying down a strong foundation of professionalism.

DBT Next Steps individual sessions and skills-training group (as well as other clinic appointments and vocational rehabilitation or employment services appointments) are opportunities to practice professional behavior. That way, you can receive feedback where there are no big or long-lasting consequences. So, practice professionalism in all sessions (except for times you and your individual therapist agree that you have a different session agenda).

DBT Next Steps clients and therapists have generated the following list of professional behaviors for group and individual sessions:

✓ Be prepared.
   - Have assignments done.
   - Have materials at hand.
   - Have reading done.
   - Be ready for good news, check in . . .
   - Complete the Diary Card and have it on hand.
   - Review new material ahead of time.
   - Set your phone to vibrate or off.

✓ Pay attention (or at least appear to).

✓ Let someone else finish their thought.

✓ Reinforce your boss or teacher.

✓ Emphasize GIVE skills.

✓ When speaking, manage your time effectively.

✓ Be on time or early.

✓ If missing or late, give notice.

✓ Come back from breaks on time.

✓ Use restroom before sessions.

✓ Keep contributions pertinent.

✓ Stay away from your phone.

✓ Get coaching ahead of time if needed.

✓ Arrive and remain regulated.

✓ Be One-Mindful to the task at hand.

✓ Reinforce your peers.

✓ Do what you say you will do.

✓ Reinforce when you use DEAR MAN.

✓ Dress appropriately, as you would if going to work or school to meet your teacher (you may want to dress for the job you want, rather than the job you have).

✓ Communicate in a way that is reinforcing (figure out what that is without asking).

✓ Communicate problems (e.g., missing or uncompleted assignments or Diary Cards) proactively *and* in a way that minimizes the burden on the other person.

✓ Be careful about off-topic comments or jokes to be sure they don't throw off the conversation.

✓ Other behaviors:

DBT-ACES Requirements toward the Recovery Goals

DBT-ACES is a comprehensive year of treatment following Standard DBT that includes all of the components of DBT Next Steps. A comprehensive DBT-ACES program has three requirements:

1. *Normative Productive Activity:* This is the requirement of being out of the house doing structured, scheduled, social planned activities.

2. *Career Development:* This is the set of activities you need to pursue to plan, train for, and carry out the career to which you aspire. These include work, school, internships, self-employment, meeting with mentors and clients, etc.

3. *Work as Therapy:* This is standard, competitive work (i.e., reported to the government by your employer) we ask you to practice during DBT-ACES so you are ready to effectively find and maintain any job until (inevitably) the time comes when you lose a job, move to a new town, or need to quickly find a new job.

To stay on track during a 6-month DBT-ACES program, you need to:

1. Continue no suicidal behaviors nor significant therapy-interfering behaviors.

2. *Normative Productive Activity:* Throughout DBT-ACES, maintain 20 hours/week of normative productive activity.

3. *Career Development:*

   - By the end of 2 months into DBT-ACES, maintain Career Development activities 10 hours/ week.

   - By the end of 4 months into DBT-ACES, maintain Career Development activities 20 hours/ week.

4. *Work as Therapy:* During the course of Standard DBT and/or DBT-ACES, you are required to work 10 hours/week at a Work as Therapy job for 6 months. This job must start by the end of 2 months into DBT-ACES.

Due dates for deadlines are always the beginning of the first DBT-ACES group of the month of the deadline (e.g., the 4-month deadline is the first group of the fifth month).

My 2-month date is: _____/_____   My 4-month date is: _____/_____

(continued)

To stay on track during a 12-month DBT-ACES program, you need to:

1. Continue no suicidal behaviors nor significant therapy-interfering behaviors.
2. *Normative Productive Activity:* Throughout DBT-ACES, maintain 20 hours/week of normative productive activity.
3. *Career Development:*
   - By the end of 4 months into DBT-ACES, maintain Career Development activities 10 hours/week.
   - By the end of 8 months into DBT-ACES, maintain Career Development activities 20 hours/week.
4. *Work as Therapy:* During the course of Standard DBT and/or DBT-ACES, you are required to work 10 hours/week at a Work as Therapy job for 6 months. This job must start by the end of 4 months into DBT-ACES.

Due dates for deadlines are always the beginning of the first DBT-ACES group of the month of the deadline (e.g., the 4-month deadline is the first group of the fifth month).

My 4-month date is: _____/_____   My 8-month date is: _____/_____

Once you have reached a deadline, you must maintain that level. If you do not meet it for 4 weeks in a row, you will be suspended from DBT-ACES until you do. As soon as you meet the requirement for 1 week, you will come back to DBT-ACES as soon as possible and still receive the remaining months of therapy in your 6- or 12-month DBT-ACES agreement (i.e., a total of either 6 or 12 months).

- We recommend (but do not require) that you tie your Work as Therapy requirement to Career Development by finding work that serves your career goal directly or allows you to save for something that does (e.g., a car). Or use the money to do something that makes you happy (e.g., take a vacation).
- Work as Therapy counts as hours toward Normative Productive Activities as well as Career Development Activities.
- Career Development Activities also count toward Normative Productive Activities.
- Diary Cards and Self-Assessment of Recovery Goals forms and other materials can be found on the Resources page at www.dbtnextsteps.com.

DBT Next Steps Check-In Long Form with Instructions

Name: _____ Date: _____

Please prepare a new sheet each week—*in writing* unless you are able to present verbally without pauses.

My Ambition (what I am passionate to achieve as a permanent change in my life; not the means to an end but an end in itself; this ambition doesn't change week to week—unless it is achieved):

Last week's *Action Step(s)* toward my ambition—what I did between last week's and this week's group:

Last week's *Employment Step(s)* toward my next deadline of _____ hours of Career Activities or work as therapy on _____/_____/

*_Progress_ (Note: First describe all parts of the Action Step(s) completed, then describe any part not completed. Avoid judgment in words, voice tone, and mental voice tone.)

(continued)

_____

*Group focus is on giving positive reinforcement (use observation skills to determine what reinforces).

_____

One *effective thing* I did to complete my Action/Employment Step(s) this week was . . .

(Describe *how you achieved your Action Step(s)* not restating your progress. Focus on what skills, strategies, or reinforcement you used to increase commitment, willingness, and to get moving.)

If not all completed, one *way I avoided* completing my Action/Employment Step(s) this week was . . .

(Describe what interfered with your step(s) such as thoughts, decisions, emotions, or actions.)

**One way I will *prevent this avoidance* behavior in the future is . . .

(Describe an effective skill, strategy, reinforcement, or mindset you can use instead of avoiding.)

One *emotion* I observed while working on my Action Step(s) was _____.

Emotions *are* joy, pride, love, happiness, contentment, sadness, desolation, disappointment, fear, panic, anxiety, anger, frustration, irritation, annoyance, shame, embarrassment, guilt, envy, etc. Emotions *are not* a thought, urge, or physical or cognitive state (e.g., confused, overwhelmed, stressed out, hopeless, tired). (The emotion doesn't have to be caused by or related to the Action Step.)

(continued)

**My *Action Step(s)* for next week will be . . .

(Describe *specifically* so it is clear when it has been completed and be sure that there is a *>50% chance* of completing it. You may want to keep with a step until you can do it reliably, increase or decrease the frequency or difficulty of the previous step, or choose a different step. Goal = effectiveness.)

**My *Employment Step(s)* for next week will be . . . (Come up with this in advance with your therapist.)

**Group focus is on understanding the nature of the problem, validating the difficulty of the problem, and problem solving and troubleshooting the plan (as needed) to learn by coaching each other.

DBT Next Steps Check-In Short Form

Name: _____ Date: _____

Please prepare a new sheet each week. Prepare it in writing unless able to present verbally without pause.

My Ambition:

Last week's *Action Step(s)* toward my ambition:

Last week's *Employment Step(s)* toward my next deadline of _____ hours of Career Activities or Work as Therapy on _____/_____/_____:

*Progress:

One *effective thing* I did to complete my Action/Employment Step(s) this week was . . .

(continued)

_____
*Group focus is on giving positive reinforcement (use observation skills to determine what reinforces).

If not all completed, one *way I avoided* completing my Action/Employment Step(s) this week was . . .

**One way I will *prevent this avoidance* behavior in the future is . . .

One *emotion* I observed while working on my Action Step(s) was . . .

**My *Action Step(s)* for next week will be . . .

**My *Employment Step(s)* for next week will be . . .

**Group focus is on understanding the nature of the problem, validating the difficulty of the problem, and problem solving and troubleshooting the plan (as needed) to learn by coaching each other.

Examples of Effective Behaviors and Ways to Prevent Avoidance

Effective Behaviors

- Break down Action Steps.
- Compare Action Step with worse tasks.
- Get on it right away.
- Persist.
- Opposite to emotion action.
- Schedule it.
- Focus on goal.
- Take materials with me.
- PLEASE skills first.
- Attend to what I like about it.
- Set up a reward for doing it.
- Pros and cons.
- Decide not to give up.
- Action Step is something I like.
- Make a public commitment.
- Take advantage of the moment.
- Pace myself.
- Fit into spare time.
- Be realistic.
- Share my success.
- Make relevant to the teaching in class.
- Want to do it so I'm prepared/can relax.
- Radical acceptance.
- Be excited/motivated for being done.
- Stay focused.
- Be effective.
- I just have to do it.
- Went through the motions until I got interested.
- Practice being open to hope.
- Wrote a script.
- Want to be with people who are into it.
- Problem-solve.
- Put things where I can see them.
- Use deadline.
- Make it fun.
- Take a positive problem-solving stance.
- Be aware of the consequences of not doing it.
- Use Wise Mind.
- Go with a group.
- Take every invitation.
- Do it in the morning (i.e., when it's a better time).
- Set alarm.
- Shape myself into it.
- Make public commitment early in the week.
- Make a contribution out of it.
- Cope ahead of time.
- One mindful.
- Stay with picture of success.
- Meet my responsibilities.
- I'm on a mission.
- No reason why I can't do this.
- Organize things first.
- Find inspiration.
- Work to calm down.
- Go with willingness.
- Have a reminder.

(continued)

Effective Behaviors *(continued)*

- Focused on what I knew I could do.
- Let go of worries about the future.

- Responded to an invitation.
- Followed my duty/responsibilities.

Avoidance Behaviors

- Prioritize other things.
- Willfulness.
- Pain interfered.
- Negative self-talk.
- Let other Action Steps wear me out.
- Tell myself there is no time.
- Procrastinated.
- Don't want to do it.
- Lost interest.
- Think "too big a task," so don't start.

- Give in to fear.
- Forget.
- Overambitious.
- Go with your depression.
- Busy with something I prefer.
- Was not clear on my Action Step.
- Lost my thunder.
- Told myself it wasn't fair.
- Chose the wrong Action Step.
- Bit off more than I could chew.

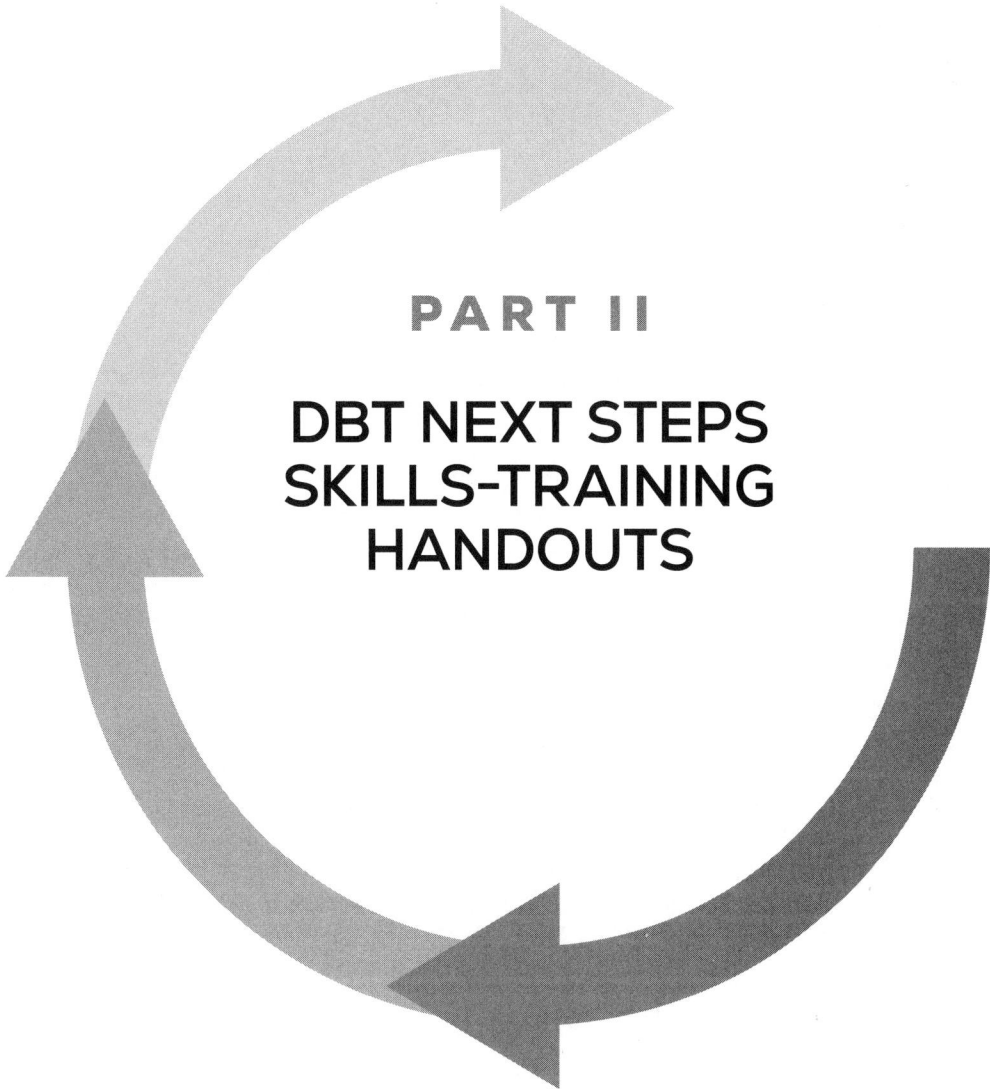

PART II

DBT NEXT STEPS SKILLS-TRAINING HANDOUTS

Perfectionism versus Reinforcement

Week	Date	Topic	Homework
1		Perfectionism versus High Achievement	• Perfectionism Worksheet*
2		High Achievement versus Being Average	• Practicing High Achievement and Being Average
3		Learn the basics of positive and negative reinforcement.	• OPTIONAL: Read Chapters 1 and 2 in *Don't Shoot the Dog* and complete answers to questions in the worksheets. • Try reinforcing someone or yourself.
4		Untraining—Stopping and Replacing Problem Behavior	• OPTIONAL: Read Chapter 4 in *Don't Shoot the Dog*. • Complete untraining thought exercise. • Complete Self-Assessment of Recovery Goals to see how you are doing.

This module is based on a wonderful book, *Don't Shoot the Dog* by Karen Pryor (2018). We recommend that you find a copy and read as much of it as you can during this module. You may also want to watch videos of clicker training or listen to the *Hidden Brain* podcast "When Everything Clicks: The Power of Judgment-Free Learning" (Schmidt et al., 2018).

---

*This assignment involves a discussion with your individual therapist. Let your individual therapist know about the assignment at the beginning of session or ahead of time so you have time to discuss.

Week 1: Perfectionism versus High Achievement

Perfectionism is a key example of being nondialectical and is often much more problematic than you realize. Here are some standard characteristics of perfectionists.

Check each that applies to you:

☐ Fear of failure — Perfectionists often equate failure to achieve their goals with a lack of personal worth or value.

☐ Fear of making mistakes — Perfectionists often equate mistakes with failure. In orienting their lives around avoiding mistakes, perfectionists miss opportunities to learn and grow.

☐ Fear of disapproval — If they let others see their flaws, perfectionists often fear that they will no longer be accepted. Trying to be perfect is a way of trying to protect themselves from criticism, rejection, or disapproval.

☐ Hiding or avoiding mistakes — Perfectionists may avoid letting others see their mistakes, not realizing self-disclosure allows others to perceive them as more human and thus more likable.

☐ All-or-nothing thinking — Perfectionists frequently believe that they are worthless if their accomplishments are not perfect. Perfectionists have difficulty seeing situations in perspective. For example, a straight "A" student who receives a "B" might believe "I am a total failure."

☐ Catastrophizing — Perfectionists often believe that if they stumble, this is the beginning of a tumble down to total destruction. This leads to panic and giving up. This does lead to at least minor destruction and serves as evidence for the catastrophe (despite the illogic).

☐ Overemphasis on "shoulds" — Perfectionists' lives are often structured by an endless list of "shoulds" that serve as rigid rules for how their lives must be led. With such an overemphasis on shoulds, perfectionists rarely take into account their own wants and desires.

☐ Believing that others are successful — Perfectionists tend to perceive others as achieving success with a minimum of effort, few errors, little emotional stress, and maximum self-confidence. At the same time, perfectionists view their own efforts as unending and forever inadequate.

☐ Discounting — Perfectionists tend to ignore, argue with, or otherwise discount feedback that is positive or encouraging and focus tremendous attention on any critical or negative feedback.

(continued)

☐ Defensiveness — Perfectionists tend to anticipate or fear disapproval and rejection from those around them. Given such fear, perfectionists may react defensively to criticism, which frustrates and alienates others.

☐ Applying perfectionism to others — Without realizing it, perfectionists may also apply unrealistic high standards to others, becoming critical and demanding of them. Thus, perfectionists have difficulty being close to people and have less than satisfactory interpersonal relationships.

Other patterns you have noticed in yourself or other perfectionists:

One Middle Road: High Achievement

In contrast to perfectionism, high achievement is dialectical—capturing the high standards of perfectionists, and the difficulties and complexities of life that make things difficult.

Do you have characteristics of a high achiever? Check each that applies to you:

☐ High achievers set their goals based on their own wants and desires, rather than primarily in response to external expectations (i.e., they balance wants and shoulds).

☐ High achievers' goals are realistic, internal, and potentially attainable.

☐ High achievers' goals are just one step beyond what they have already accomplished.

☐ High achievers take pleasure in the process of achieving the task, not just the end result.

☐ High achievers can visualize their goals as a series of steps one after another leading to a successful end result. They can also visualize themselves coping with each step and succeeding in the end—despite setbacks.

☐ High achievers are effective troubleshooters—they not only have a Plan B, they also have developed Plans C, D, and E as needed. High achievers are not stuck on Plan A; they are willing to jump to B or C when that is more effective.

☐ High achievers encourage and reward themselves for steps along the process, not just for the final goal or end result. They reinforce themselves for effort even (or especially) when things are not working out in the moment.

☐ When high achievers experience disapproval or failure, their reactions are generally limited to specific situations rather than generalized to their entire self-worth (i.e., they don't catastrophize).

☐ High achievers recognize when they need help and ask for it from others. But they don't give control or responsibility for the problem to the other person. They get advice or a leg up and then keep going on their own.

Other high achiever characteristics:

Week 1 Assignment:
Exploring High Achievement over Perfectionism

1. Review your symptoms of perfectionism and high achievement from the lists above in the week 1 materials. Read them again.

Describe what being a high achiever and perfectionist means specifically for you:

Being a High Achiever: What does this look like? List what you would do . . .

_____

_____

_____

_____

_____

_____

Being a Perfectionist: What does this look like? List what you would do . . .

_____

_____

_____

_____

_____

_____

2. Write down the personal pros and cons* of being a high achiever versus attempting to be perfect:

Being a High Achiever: PROS

_____

_____

_____

_____

_____

Being a Perfectionist: PROS

_____

_____

_____

_____

_____

Being a High Achiever: CONS

_____

_____

_____

_____

_____

_____

Being a Perfectionist: CONS

_____

_____

_____

_____

_____

_____

*Remember to consider the short-term AND long-term pros and cons.

Why Be a High Achiever (and Not a Perfectionist)?

Copying from the responses to Question 2 in the Week 1 Assignment, make a list of the PROS of being a high achiever and the CONS of being a perfectionist (the upper left and lower right of the table). This is a single list of all the reasons to move toward being a high achiever. Take a picture or make a copy of this list, place it somewhere convenient, and use it to stick with the goal of becoming a high achiever (even when you have perfectionist urges).

_____

_____

_____

_____

_____

_____

_____

_____

_____

_____

_____

3. Give yourself credit for small accomplishments every day this week.

Today, I accomplished:

Monday	
Tuesday	
Wednesday	
Thursday	
Friday	
Saturday	
Sunday	

(continued)

4. Observe and describe past mistakes and failures and figure out how you overcame them and moved forward (give at least two examples).

5. Practice radical acceptance of your strengths and weaknesses, and your accomplishments and failures, by writing five acceptance (not approval) statements about yourself below.

   a.

   b.

   c.

   d.

   e.

6. In a sentence written to yourself, *give yourself permission to make mistakes.* Practice saying this sentence aloud (to yourself or others) with conviction.

7. Share this completed homework with your individual therapist.

Week 2: Another Middle Road Option: Being Average

Being average is a lot better than being a perfectionist. If you don't want to be a high achiever, strive for average. Average is defined as "typical example of the group under consideration," not the low end. Thus, being average is another middle road.

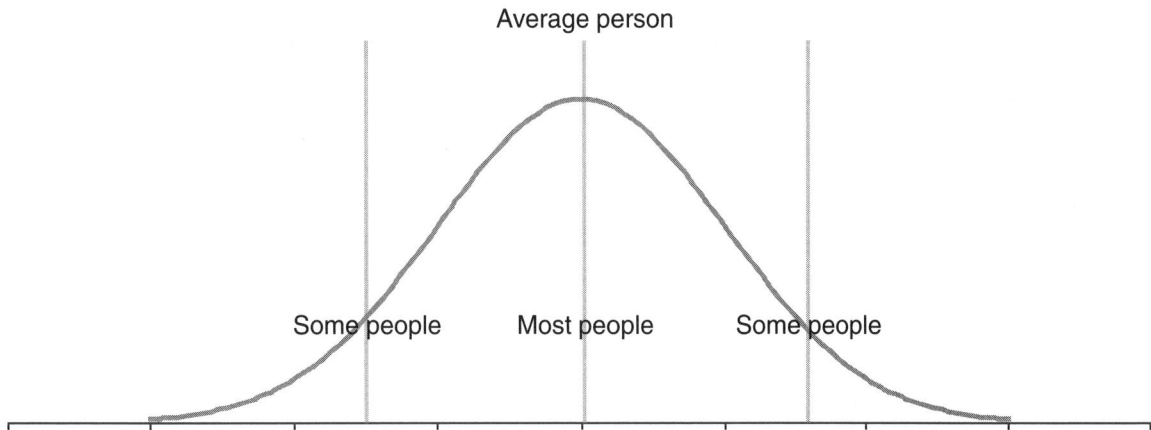

Characteristics of an average approach (check each that apply to you):

☐ Don't let someone down—but don't show initiative.

☐ Do just enough to achieve your goal (e.g., good enough grades to graduate, get an average performance evaluation with no major dings).

☐ Let someone else be the leader and relax into the role of following.

☐ Do what is asked, but nothing in addition.

☐ Do not think about tasks when you don't have to (e.g., don't schedule time to work on tasks at home, don't go out of your way to make your relationship better).

☐ When you can imagine there's a more efficient or effective way to do something, just let the idea pass without acting on it.

Remember: One does not need to be a high achiever in everything—one can be an average employee and a high-achieving spouse or parent or vice versa.

Positive and/or effective examples of being average:

Week 2 Assignment:
Practicing Alternatives to Being a Perfectionist

1. Identify as many areas as you can in which you tend toward perfectionism:

   - Things you think you have to do right or thoughts that there is only one right way to do something

   - Expectations that everyone should like you, validate you, appreciate you

   - Expectations that you will always act appropriately

   - Tendency to quit when your performance is not perfect

(continued)

2. Choose two specific examples of perfectionism from the list above to work on this week.

   ● Perfectionist Behavior 1:

   ● Perfectionist Behavior 2:

(continued)

3. This homework asks you to practice the experience of being a "high achiever" and "average." Notice how those experiences make you feel—what you like and don't like about each one.

   a. *For Perfectionist Behavior 1:* Practice being a "high achiever." Look over the list of high-achiever behaviors and describe how they apply to this perfectionist behavior.

   b. Now practice these high-achiever strategies *consistently* all week for situations involving Perfectionist Behavior 1. When you forget, remind yourself and try again. Note your observations of the experience here.

(continued)

c. *For Perfectionist Behavior 2:* Practice being "average." Look over the list of average strategies and describe how they apply to this perfectionist behavior.

d. Now practice applying these average strategies *consistently* all week in situations related to Perfectionist Behavior 2. Do a good enough job. Note your observations of the experience here.

(continued)

4. Choose one day when you decide to have no expectations. Don't expect people to be friendly—when they are not, you won't be surprised or bothered; if they are, you'll be delighted. Don't expect your day to be problem-free. Instead, as problems come up, say to yourself "Ah, another hurdle to overcome."

   a. Rather than fighting against life—dance with it.

   b. If you notice that you're having an expectation, let go of it and return to having no expectations.

      • Observations of things you noticed yourself expecting:

      • Observations about the experience of not expecting anything:

Week 3: The Basics of Reinforcement

1. What is reinforcement? What's the point? How is it different from a reward?

2. What is positive reinforcement?
   "Positive reinforcement is anything which, occurring in conjunction with an act, tends to increase the probability that the act will occur again" (Pryor, 2018, p. 1). What does this mean?

   What are some examples of positive reinforcement?

3. What is negative reinforcement? How is it different from punishment?
   "Negative reinforcement is something a subject will work to avoid. . . . Punishment comes after a behavior it is meant to affect. Thus you can't avoid receiving a punishment by changing your mind, or your actions, since the misbehavior has already happened. . . . Negative reinforcement, on the other hand, may be halted or avoided by changing behavior right now" (Pryor, 2018, p. 1). So, what does this mean?

   What are some examples of negative reinforcement?

(continued)

4. Who decides what is reinforcing, and how do you know if you reinforced it?

   How does this law of behavior apply to your examples above?

5. Reinforcement is information—it tells the subject *exactly* what it is you like.

   If you time it wrong, you give the wrong information!

   • If you give positives in a debriefing after a soccer game or ballet recital, you reinforce being part of the group and playing or dancing in general. You do not reinforce the specific moves you want to see, even if you talk about them.

   • What would you have to do to reinforce the exact movements/kicks/timing you wanted?

6. Big reinforcers need smaller reinforcers that add up to the big one (e.g., points, gold stars, pennies) and can only be used with *agreement* of the subject. However, agreement is often the least helpful thing to get! Why?

7. Note, you have to be sure not to reinforce when the behavior doesn't occur or you will confuse your subject!

Schedules of Reinforcement

Schedule of reinforcement	Definition	When to use	Examples	Examples that relate to you
Continuous reinforcement	Every instance of a designated response is reinforced.	Often used to shape and establish a behavior.	Getting a soda every time you put money in a vending machine.	
Intermittent reinforcement	A designated response is reinforced only some of the time.	Tends to generate a steadier response and greater resistance to extinction.	Receiving verbal praise from your boss when you complete some of your reports on time. Other reports get no response.	
Fixed ratio	Reinforcer is given after a fixed number of responses.	Gets a fast response until quota is reached, then pause.	Salesperson receives a bonus for every 5 cars sold.	
Variable ratio	Reinforcer is given after a variable number of responses.	Gets high and steady rate of response as long as reinforcer is given just often enough.	Slot machine pays off once every 10 tries *on average* (number between each payoff varies, but averages to 10).	
Fixed interval	Reinforcer is given for the first response that occurs after a fixed time has elapsed.	Increases right before reinforcer, if action required, and pause after.	Paycheck every 2 weeks or morphine drip every 4 hours.	
Variable interval	Reinforcer is given for the first response after a variable time has elapsed.	Steady response until right after reinforcer when expected delay leads to pause.	Surfer waits for a surf-able wave that varies widely but comes *on average* every 15 minutes.	

35

Other Reinforcement Concepts

Other concepts	Definition	When to use	Examples	Examples that relate to you
"Slow start" problem (a.k.a. delayed start of long-duration behavior)	Putting off starting a behavior or task when the schedule of reinforcement is longer (i.e., takes longer to get reinforced).	—	Putting off taking down the Christmas lights.	
Superstitious behavior	Occurs when the delivery of a reinforcer or punisher occurs close together in time with an independent behavior, and the behavior is accidentally reinforced or punished.	—	You eat a banana for breakfast right before a successful job interview. You then start eating bananas before important things in your life. Or, you believe one of your t-shirts is your lucky fishing shirt.	
Noncontingent reinforcement	Giving reinforcement independent of the target behavior.	To improve morale or the relationship, or create surprise or interest.	Lots of positive reinforcement offered to babies and new romance, or giving a bored dolphin a bucket of fish for nothing.	
Incompatible behavior	A desired behavior that cannot occur at the same time as a behavior you don't want.	Can't reinforce less of a behavior, so provides what to reinforce.	Reinforcing a soft voice to get less yelling.	

36

From *DBT Next Steps Skills Handouts: Building a Life Worth Living*, by Katherine Anne Comtois, Adam Carmel, and Marsha M. Linehan. Copyright © 2025 The Guilford Press. Permission to photocopy this material or download it from the epdf is granted to purchasers of this book for personal use or use with clients; see copyright page for details.

Practicing Reinforcement

1. What are specific behaviors one could reinforce? Let's troubleshoot them.

2. What are possible reinforcers for other people? Note, big reinforcers need smaller reinforcers that add up to the big one (e.g., points, gold stars, pennies). Let's troubleshoot them.

Positive reinforcers that are small and easy to do over and over (i.e., things you can add)	Negative reinforcers that are small and easy to do over and over (i.e., things you can stop)	Positive reinforcements that are too big to do often

Week 3 Assignment: Practicing Reinforcement

1. OPTIONAL: Read Chapters 1 and 2 in *Don't Shoot the Dog* (Pryor, 2018), listen to the *Hidden Brain* podcast on clicker training (Schmidt et al., 2018), and watch clicker-training videos.

2. What is a behavior you would like *someone else* to do more of? (If it is a behavior you want to decrease, hold off on it until next week or go with an incompatible behavior you could increase that would replace what you want to decrease.)

3. What are some possible reinforcers for the behavior?

Positive reinforcers that are small and easy to do over and over (i.e., things you can add)	Negative reinforcers that are small and easy to do over and over (i.e., things you can stop)	Positive reinforcements that are too big to do often

(continued)

4. Describe a reinforcement schedule to increase this behavior and troubleshoot it.

5. *Switching to yourself,* what is a behavior you would like to increase/be more effective at/do more of? (If it is a behavior you want to decrease, think of an incompatible behavior you could increase that would automatically replace it.)

(continued)

6. What are some reinforcers for you?

Positive reinforcers that are small and easy to do over and over (i.e., things you can add)	Negative reinforcers that are small and easy to do over and over (i.e., things you can stop)	Positive reinforcements that are too big to do often

7. Describe a reinforcement schedule to increase this behavior and troubleshoot it.

(continued)

8. Pick *either* the other person *or* yourself, and try your plan this week.

9. Afterward, describe what you ended up doing: (a) Who were you reinforcing, (b) what behavior did you decide to increase, (c) what did the reinforcer end up being, (d) how did you do it?

10. Describe the results: Did anything change? As you expected? Did the desired behavior occur? Was the reinforcer actually provided quickly after the desired behavior occurred? What did you notice about your response to this exercise?

Week 4: Untraining or Making It Stop!

In Chapter 4 of *Don't Shoot the Dog* (Pryor, 2018), there are eight methods to untrain a behavior—a.k.a. make it stop. Half are considered the "bad fairies"—they work but have costs. Half are the "good fairies"—they work with few costs, but take time and effort to achieve.

Exercise

1. As a group, let's pick two behaviors we don't like and would like to untrain.
2. Everyone pick a "good fairy" and/or a "bad fairy" method.
3. Leader or client, read a summary of each method and apply it to the examples.
4. Discuss how to apply the methods to untraining other behaviors we don't like.

	1st behavior to untrain	2nd behavior to untrain
Bad Fairies		
Method 1: Shoot the dog		
Method 2: Punishment		
Method 3: Negative reinforcement		
Method 4: Extinction		

(continued)

	1st behavior to untrain	2nd behavior to untrain
Good Fairies		
Method 5: Train an incompatible behavior		
Method 6: Put the behavior on cue		
Method 7: Shape the absence of the behavior		
Method 8: Change the motivation		

Week 4 Assignment: Untraining Behavior

1. OPTIONAL: Read Chapters 3 and 4 in *Don't Shoot the Dog* (Pryor, 2018).

2. Thought exercise: Consider how you could untrain a behavior you don't like.

<u>Problem behavior</u>: What does someone (or a pet) do that is driving you nuts or wearing you out? *Be sure to choose someone else's behavior for this assignment.*

<u>Give an example of how to apply each method to untraining this problem behavior based on the class discussion</u>: *Some methods will work more effectively than others with a given problem. Be creative, flexible, and maybe a little silly in your examples.*

	Example applied to your situation
Bad Fairies	
Method 1: Shoot the dog	
Method 2: Punishment	

(continued)

	Example applied to your situation
Method 3: Negative reinforcement	
Method 4: Extinction	
Good Fairies	
Method 5: Train an incompatible behavior	
Method 6: Put the behavior on cue	
Method 7: Shape the absence of the behavior	
Method 8: Change the motivation	

Self-Assessment of DBT Next Steps Recovery Goals

Name:	Months into DBT Next Steps:	Date:

1. Please note how far you have come on each of these Recovery Goals that are the focus of DBT Next Steps on the following scale and check which Recovery Goals you are currently working on with your individual therapist.

0 = Not thought about it or talked about it

1 = Thought or talked about it, no action, don't want to

2 = Thought or talked about it, no action, want to

3 = Tried to do/get it but couldn't

4 = Trying to do it, can do/have it, once or twice

5 = Trying to do it, can do/have it, not reliably

6 = Do/have this reliably, still have problems being effective

7 = Do/have this reliably, this problem is essentially solved

Recovery Goals	Number	✓ if current target
Living Wage Employment and Off Psychiatric Disability		
Choose a career path to living wage employment knowing its fit with your Wise Mind values and talents as well as the practical issues of pay, health insurance, leave and retirement benefits, hours, shift times, required training or certification, and routes to advancement.		
Demonstrate capability to financially support yourself (and your family) in your chosen career without psychiatric disability payments or partner's/family's income.		
Demonstrate capability to financially support yourself (and your family) in at least one fallback job without psychiatric disability payments or partner's/family's income (if needed).		
Sufficient health insurance to maintain health care and medications.		
Better than 90% follow-through at work on attendance, being on time, appropriate dress and manner, following directions, and job tasks.		

(continued)

Recovery Goals	Number	✓ if current target
Interpersonal Proficiency		
Interpersonally easy to work/be with—even with difficult people and during stressful times.		
Demonstrate capability to regulate emotional expression and actions, and find Wise Mind in all interpersonal situations—even with difficult people and during stressful times.		
Know your Wise Mind personal limits and act on them with yourself, employer, friends, family, colleagues, and members of your community.		
Receive praise, raises, promotions, and offers for more desirable jobs and roles within your community.		
Life Outside Work *(Note: These categories are expected to overlap.)*		
Have at least a couple of local and/or long-distance friends whose values align with yours.		
Have at least one person or group for casual interactions (e.g., lunchroom, church, coffee, movie, book club, volunteer organization).		
Have at least one close support with whom you experience intimacy and discuss private issues (who is not your therapist).		
Have at least one local person or group that would notice you were not around and would take action to find you.		
Be an active member of an organized recreational activity that is either fun or meaningful and not related to mental health (e.g., volunteer organization, church, sports teams, Spanish lessons, ballroom dancing).		
Disengage from relationships with family members that are ineffective or destructive.		
Disengage or end friendships that are ineffective or destructive.		
Choose relationships based on evidence that they are compatible with your lifestyle, needs, and values.		
Take steps to find an effective and rewarding romantic relationship (if desired).		

(continued)

Recovery Goals	Number	✓ if current target
Emotional Proficiency		
Able to experience negative emotions building, staying, and falling mindfully—not avoiding, rushing them along, or mentally moving into a different moment.		
Able to experience positive emotions building, staying, and falling mindfully—not avoiding, rushing them along, or mentally moving into a different moment.		
Able to reduce problematic emotions effectively and fast enough to prevent them from leading to problems.		
Self-Management		
Have an effective method for managing your monthly budget and one-time expenses (e.g., new tires) so you stay within your income.		
Sufficient emergency fund savings to cover 3 months of living expenses in case you lose your job.		
Have an effective method of savings for things you would enjoy.		
Have an effective method for getting out of debt/getting debt to a reasonable level.		
Have an effective method for managing your time that means spending your time in line with your Wise Mind values.		
Have an effective method for managing your time that gets key things done on time.		
Have an effective method for managing your time that balances work, leisure, household, and downtime.		
Have an effective method of preventing illness and psychiatric symptoms from impacting your functioning.		
Have an effective method of managing chronic illness or pain to minimize its impact on your quality of life.		

(continued)

2. One of the characteristics of a life worth living outside of mental health is significant responsibilities that require time, timeliness, follow-through, patience, interest, creativity, etc. These responsibilities tend to benefit one's mental health. We'd like to know what responsibilities you have and whether they are something established that isn't requiring a lot of effort or something that you are starting to work on and requires significant attention.

List people, places, and things that I am responsible for/to:	✓ the appropriate box	
	Established/ easy	Just starting/ challenging

Establishing and Re-Evaluating Relationships

Week	Date	Topic	Assignments (due the following week)
1		Observing and Describing Current and Ideal Maps of My Community	• Complete Current and Ideal Maps.
2		Establishing New Relationships	• Complete Diving In Assignment.
3		Re-establishing Old Relationships	• Observe and describe key aspects of two relationships.
4		Toning Down and Stopping GIVE Skills	• Practice casual conversation. • Practice STOP skills.

Week 1: Developing Accurate and Ideal Maps of My Community

People and Organizations Who Can Be in Your Community: friends, work, school, volunteer organization, political movement, online community, local government, community or neighborhood group, spiritual or religious organization, social club, sports team or club, health club, 12-step group, nonmental health support group, weight-loss program, friendship network, best friend, romantic partner, family of origin, children, pen pal, etc.

Active and Effective Participation in Your Community:

- You are a desired member of this community, to which you value and contribute, <u>and</u>
- Your absence causes expressions of interest or concern.

Please list the types of communities in which you are already an active and effective participant:

Please list the types of communities in which you would like to become an active and effective participant during the next 5 years:

Community Mapping

Look at the community map on p. 57, the Sample Community Map, and the completed example included in Appendix 4.

It is arranged as concentric shapes from the center heart for those closest to you through more casual relationships, to an outer circle of people you would like out of your life.

Let's play around with this sample map. Start by putting people or categories of people onto the map as they are or as you'd like them to be. Consider the following:

- Who goes in the center heart? Anyone? Many people? One or two people?
- If you aren't sure of specific people, put in a label (e.g., if you don't have a best friend but want one, put "best friend" on the map)
- Work on being nonjudgmental. Perhaps you are an extrovert, and there are many people who are key people or center heart people? Maybe you are an introvert, and you have few people close to you on your map and like it that way? Maybe somewhere in between . . .
- Who is in your community who might be more effectively left out of it? All the way out of it? Kept at a more casual level?
- Who might have drifted out or been pushed out who might do better back in the community? How close should they be?
- There is no right and wrong map per se. The key is a map that reflects your Wise Mind—not only your Reason or Emotion Mind about what you can or should have.

Here are some suggestions of people to include (or actions to take) from the DBT Next Steps Recovery Goals (remember, one person may serve multiple roles so you don't have to include a lot of people):

- At least a couple of local and/or long-distance friends whose values align with yours
- At least one person or group for casual interactions (e.g., lunchroom, church, coffee, movie, book club, volunteer organization)
- At least one close support with whom you experience intimacy and discuss private issues (someone who is not your therapist)
- At least one local person or group that would notice you were not around and would take action to find you
- An effective and rewarding romantic relationship (if desired)
- Select an organized recreational activity that is either fun or meaningful and not related to mental health (e.g., volunteer organization, church, sports teams, gym class, Spanish lessons, ballroom dancing).
- Disengage from relationships with family members that are ineffective or destructive.
- Disengage or end friendships that are ineffective or destructive.

Sample Community Map

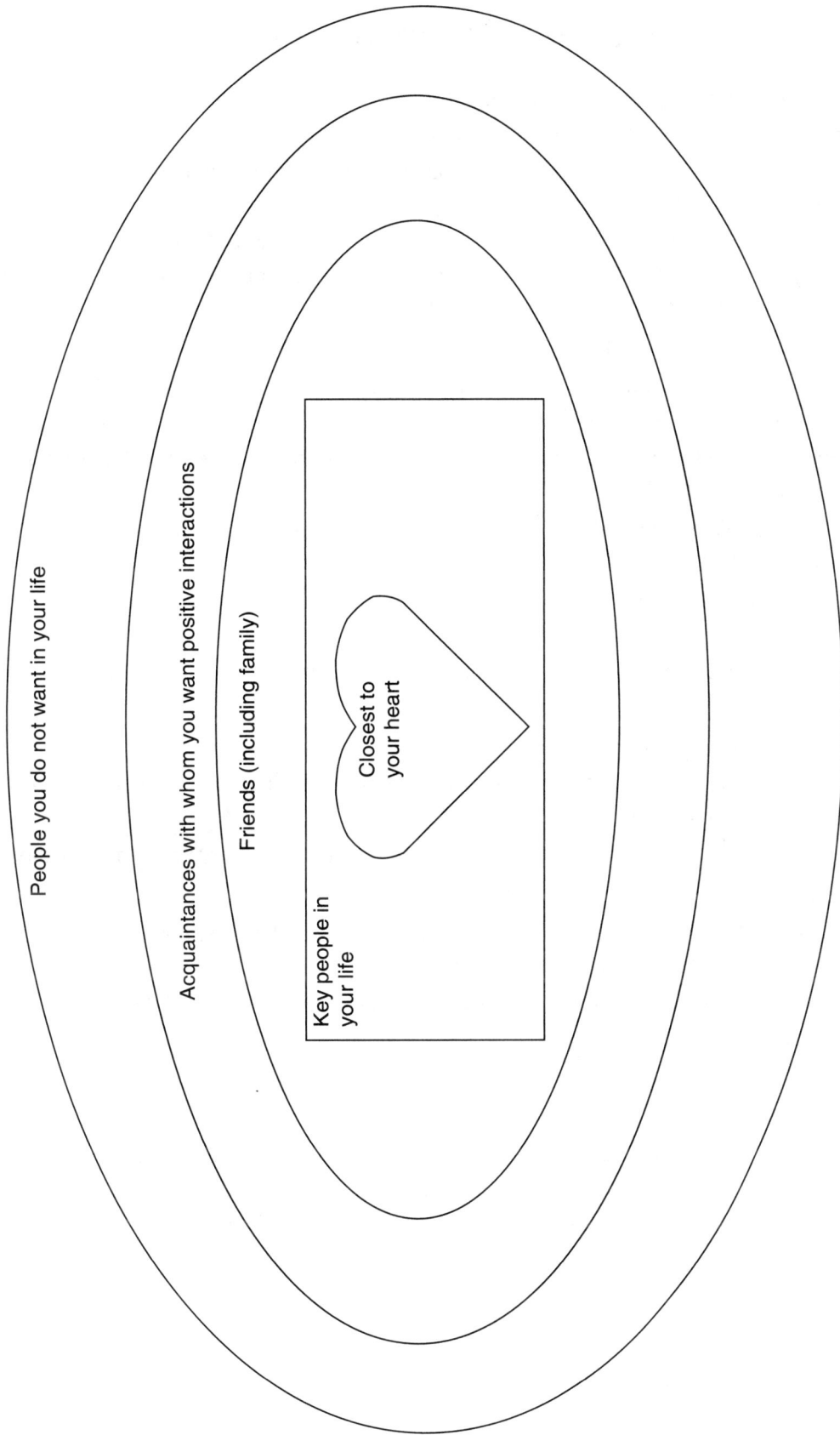

People you do not want in your life

Acquaintances with whom you want positive interactions

Friends (including family)

Key people in your life

Closest to your heart

Week 1 Assignment: Complete Maps Now and Ideal

1. Review pp. 57–58, where two maps, marked "Now" and "Ideal," appear. Your assignment this week is to thoroughly complete both of these maps.

   • You may want to use a pencil or make a couple of copies of each map before you start, so you can easily make changes or revise drafts.

   • Do not expect to do this task in one sitting. That will likely lead to Emotion Mind maps or getting stuck. Do a draft and then leave it for a day or 2. Look at the maps with a fresh eye; see what still makes sense and what to change.

2. Complete Community Map 1 (p. 57) with the people in your life NOW.

   a. Forget whether you are happy about how things are; use your Observe and Describe skills to develop an accurate picture of your community.

   b. You can put categories of people on your map (e.g., "women I work with," "neighbors," "other meet-up members," "cousins on dad's side").

3. Next, complete Community Map 2 (p. 58) based on an IDEAL world. (Think in terms of 2 or 5 or 10 years from now, if that helps.)

   a. The first step is to start fresh by putting people on the Ideal map regardless of your Now map (or the sample map).

      • Build an ideal world: Let go of what is possible, and observe and describe only what you wish for in Wise Mind.

      • Practice willingness and hopefulness.

   b. Once you have a fresh Ideal map, using Wise Mind, be sure all the people from your Now are on your Ideal map exactly where you want them.

      • Would some people be closer, others be farther out, some out of your life altogether?

      • Find a spot for everyone on the Ideal map.

      • If you just aren't sure, note those people on the edge of the paper, outside of the circles. You may need to reconsider them later.

   c. Next, again using Wise Mind, consider who might be missing from your Ideal map.

      • Where do they go?

      • Remember, you can put labels for people you don't yet know (e.g., best friend, love of my life, wife, boss, child).

4. Observe and describe the experience of making these maps. Anything surprise you? What differs between your Now and Ideal maps? Anything you notice that was effective or ineffective? Anything that helped or got in the way?

Community Map 1: Now

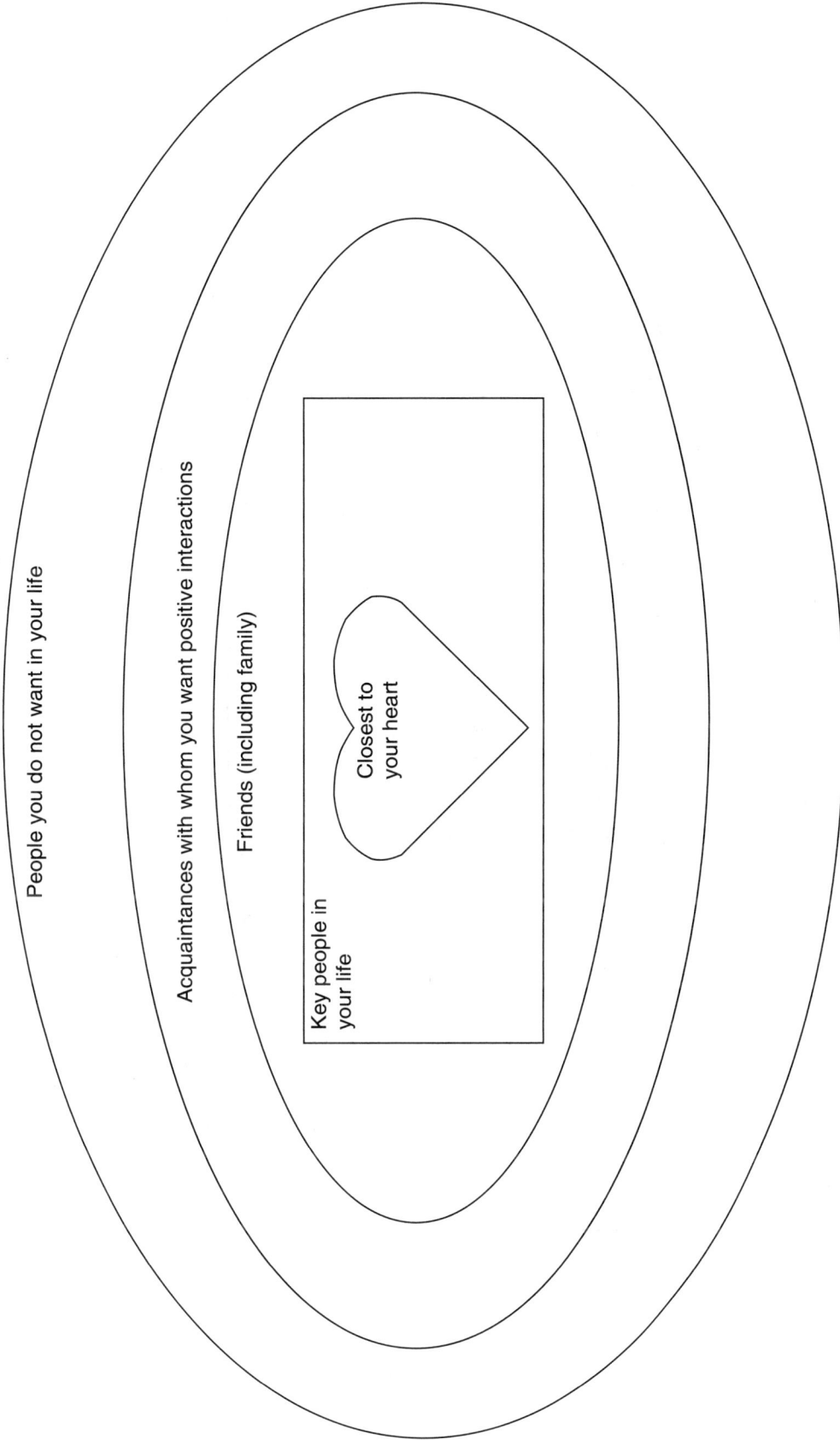

People you do not want in your life

Acquaintances with whom you want positive interactions

Friends (including family)

Key people in your life

Closest to your heart

Community Map 2: Ideal

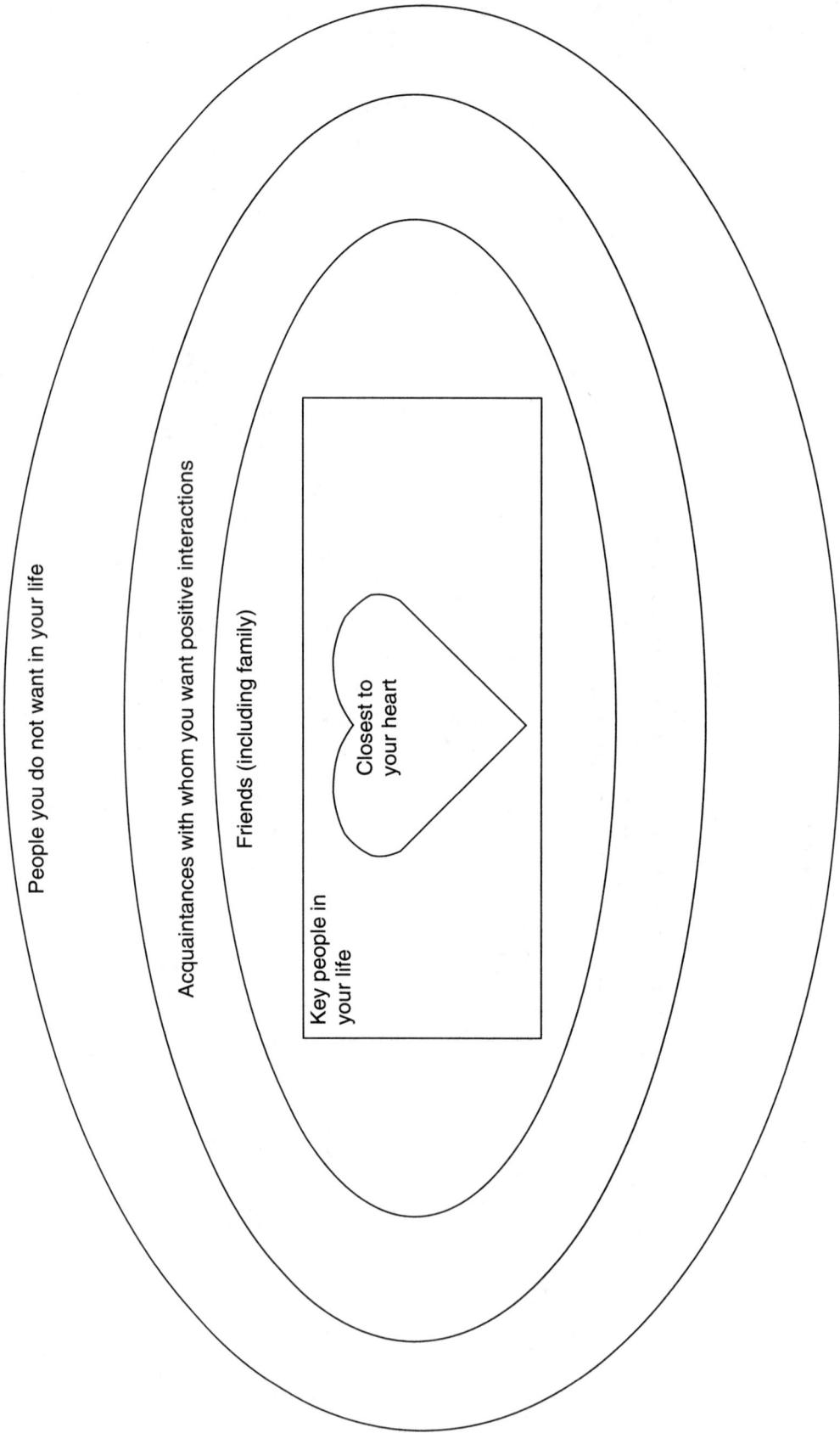

People you do not want in your life

Acquaintances with whom you want positive interactions

Friends (including family)

Key people in your life

Closest to your heart

Week 2: Diving Into New Relationships

This week, the focus is on diving into new relationships and making them work.

Preparing for Finding Satisfying Relationships:

1. Practice the Problem-Solving skill for how to meet and connect with new people. Figure out the way in which you want to handle things. Make a plan.

2. Practice Cope Ahead of Time skills for when you are with new people. Imagine using your plan for how you want to handle things. Imagine things going well. Imagine things going poorly and still being skillful.

3. Practice willingness to take on the risk of rejection to get what you want. Be willing to fall on your face and get back up. Try the Half-Smile and Willing Hands skills.

4. When not with others, work on reducing thoughts that interfere with finding ideal relationships (e.g., hopeless or helpless thoughts, self-pity, judgments).

Strategies for Finding Satisfying Relationships:

1. Go to a new place or look at the usual place with new eyes.

2. Go to the same place at the same time regularly.

3. Do something you like/value so your time is well spent, whatever happens.

4. Decide for how long you are going to throw yourself into the activity (e.g., "I'm going to this meet-up for 1 hour") and participate fully until then. When you get close to the time frame you chose, use Wise Mind to decide whether to continue.

5. Participate fully—immerse yourself. Block any thoughts about how you appear to others because those thoughts can make you miss cues and appear odd.

6. Give messages of interest: make eye contact, smile at someone, engage in small talk.

7. Use lots and lots of GIVE skills. Focus on making other people comfortable.

8. Gather information when you are around others. Observe one-mindfully and nonjudgmentally what you see and hear, what emotions you experience, what thoughts you have, and, importantly, who you prefer to be around.

9. Recognize your preferences without judging. What do you like or dislike about individuals or them collectively as a group . . . How is the experience, or isn't it a fit for you?

(continued)

10. Let go of rigid thinking (e.g., "friends should . . . ," "if I do, it looks . . . ," "that's not how it's done . . . ") and be spontaneous, without expectations, and willing.

11. Don't put all your eggs in one basket; pursue several options. Most people will not work out.

Strategies for Making Relationships Satisfying:

1. Go slowly—this isn't a race. Give yourself time to decide how much someone is a fit for you, and practice GIVE and FAST, using Wise Mind.

2. Remember, if GIVE skills attract the wrong people, switch the intensity of your communication or kindly but firmly say or show you're not interested.

3. Pursue possible relationships with an exit strategy. Meet people in a public place and for a fixed duration so you can leave easily or plan to meet again.

4. Doing something does not mean you have to make a commitment. If someone expects a commitment very soon, that is information about them.

5. If someone is not a fit, practice letting them go by your words or actions.

Week 2 Assignment:
Do One Thing Every Day toward New Relationships

Each day, do at least one Diving In activity to bring new relationships into your life: mix and match preparing, finding, and making relationships satisfying activities. Observe and describe the results as we do our Action Steps in the Check-In.

Day	What I did to make new relationships more likely	What was one effective thing I did to accomplish this?	What emotion did I observe?
Friday			
Saturday			
Sunday			

(continued)

Day	What I did to make new relationships more likely	What was one effective thing I did to accomplish this?	What emotion did I observe?
Monday			
Tuesday			
Wednesday			
Thursday			

Week 3: Re-Establishing Existing Relationships

Think of relationships that you would consider restarting or reinvigorating. Maybe you have drifted apart, are treading water, or had a falling out. Consider some examples of such people in your life (including friends, family, coworkers, social media friends, neighbors, high school buddies, soccer friends, meet-up members)?

To re-establish a relationship, the first step is to accurately and mindfully observe and describe the relationship as it stands:

- Describe what you like about the other person.

- Describe how the other person supports or validates you.

- Describe times the other person has sacrificed or stepped up for you.

- Describe what you dislike about the other person.

- Describe when the person may have disappointed or invalidated you.

(continued)

What do you remember now about your reactions?

	Emotions	Thoughts	Body sensations	Actions I took
When you were feeling really connected/having a particularly good time?				
When things were typical of how you are/were together?				
When things didn't go well between you?				

Let's practice a Wise Mind exercise to find Wise Mind about this relationship.

What do you conclude (circle your response)?　　Yes　　No　　Maybe　　Try and see

Week 3 Assignment:
Accurate Assessment of Two Relationships

Person 1: _____

• Describe whom this person is/was in your life? How did/do you know them?

• Describe what you like about the other person, how they support/ed you or validate/ed you, times they sacrificed or stepped up for you.

• Describe what you dislike about the other person, when they may have disappointed or invalidated you.

(continued)

What do you remember now about your reactions then?

	Emotions	Thoughts	Body sensations	Actions I took
When you were feeling really connected/having a particularly good time?				
When things were typical of how you are/were together?				
When things didn't go well between you?				

Practice a Wise Mind exercise to determine if this relationship makes sense to re-establish. What exercise did you practice? _____

What do you conclude (circle your response)?   Yes   No   Maybe   Try and see

(continued)

66

Person 2: _____

- Describe whom this person is/was in your life? How did/do you know them?

- Describe what you like about the other person, how they support/ed you or validate/ed you, times they sacrificed or stepped up for you.

- Describe what you dislike about the other person, when they may have disappointed or invalidated you.

(continued)

What do you remember now about your reactions then?

	Emotions	Thoughts	Body sensations	Actions I took
When you were feeling really connected/having a particularly good time?				
When things were typical of how you are/were together?				
When things didn't go well between you?				

Practice a Wise Mind exercise to determine if this relationship makes sense to re-establish. What exercise did you practice? _____

What do you conclude (circle your response)?   Yes   No   Maybe   Try and see

Week 4: Variations on GIVE:
Casual Conversation and Creating Distance

Being Casual: How to do a "toned-down" GIVE for casual conversations with new people in social or professional situations.

1. *When you arrive, scan the physical space.* That way, you can extricate yourself from conversation (to find your seat, get coffee, use the restroom, catch someone who's leaving) without breaking eye contact. Wandering eyes make you look bored, even if all you are trying to do is smoothly transition to wherever you are going next.

2. *Use eye contact.* The best way to make someone feel comfortable with you is a combination of repeated, but extremely brief, eye contact + being observed to be an effective person with an easy manner. Eye contact moves an interpersonal interaction from people in the same place to a dyad—too much at first is too intimate and intrusive, but too little indicates disinterest. Synthesis—keep adding a little over time. The brief eye contact means the person has noticed you. During the time you aren't looking at each other, they can see what you do and how you interact with others, which makes them more confident and comfortable with you. (*Note:* This can happen over 45 minutes at a meeting or over months of seeing each other at the gym or the mailboxes.)

3. *For the best conversation, start it yourself!* Nervous? Look at it this way: You are saving the person you chat up a lot of agony. The vast majority of people say they are shy in social situations. Saying something that opens the door for dialogue breaks the ice for others. This is the time to Act Interested.

4. *Too much information!* Too much too soon could overload the person or just creep them out. Given that people tend to slowly increase how much personal information they share, if you share a lot of personal information early on, others may feel you are boundary-less and be unclear how far you'll go. . . . Thus, they will back off to remain safe.

5. *Keep it light.* Light doesn't have to mean funny—many professional situations don't call for that—but a half-smile is always a good place to start. Imagine being the floater on the fishing line, not the weight; if the hook goes too low, help bring it back up. You can do this by a gentle change of topic, asking a pleasant and polite question, or talking about the weather, local sports, or the like.

6. *To end a conversation, perfect the "subtle shift."* People are afraid to move on because they don't want to appear rude to the person they're speaking with. Keep your focus on them until you are ready. Then try saying, "It's been so much fun talking to you, but I wanted to _____!" Now, smile with eye contact, then <u>quick!</u> graciously break eye contact, say/gesture goodbye, and walk to another person, leave. (If you drag out the shift or give mixed signals, they don't know what to do: Keep talking? Stop talking?)

(continued)

Learn that the opposite of GIVE . . . STOP (a different skill than the one in Distress Tolerance) is used to avoid friends, get distance from family, and prevent being asked on a date, and so on.

STOP Skills

Sharp	Unlike being Gentle, this means focusing on creative means for escaping the situation—even if they aren't entirely sincere; if you have to stay, don't judge or attack, but err on the side of directness and not pulling your punches.
Thoughtless	Unlike Validating, don't give verbal or nonverbal cues that you are in sync with the person—look blankly in their direction, but don't nod at appropriate times, maintain eye contact with something else (e.g., your glass, your phone, someone else), don't say you see their point of view even if you do.
Offended	Unlike Easy Manner, be more easily offended, don't smile, but rather express irritation—perhaps not at the person but at something in the situation, how you have a headache or so much work to do, the weather.
Preoccupied	Unlike being Interested, don't make an attempt to respond to the content of what the person is saying; talk about your own topic or just nod vaguely.

Week 4 Assignment:
Casual Conversation and Creating Distance

1. Observe and describe all of the places in which effective casual conversation is important in your life (consider work, school, where you live, friends and family events, who you interact with as the day goes along, etc.)

2. Consider each of the six casual conversation skills. Observe and describe how, when, and where they apply in your life:

   • *When you arrive, scan the physical space:*

   • *Use eye contact:*

   • *For the best conversation, start it yourself:*

(continued)

- *Too much information!:*

- *Keep it light:*

- *To end a conversation, perfect the "subtle shift":*

3. Practice using all six casual conversation skills across at least three different situations this week (i.e., not all skills in one place, but all skills at least once).

   Check off which you did at least once (full descriptions on the handout):

   ☐ When you arrive, scan the physical space.

   ☐ Use eye contact.

   ☐ For the best conversation, start it yourself!

   ☐ Too much information!

   ☐ Keep it light.

   ☐ To end a conversation, perfect the "subtle shift."

Observations about using these skills in casual conversation situations:

(continued)

STOP Skills

1. Describe what STOP skills are in your own words. What are they for?

2. *This week*, put yourself in <u>two</u> situations that *especially* call for STOP skills (e.g., talking with someone you no longer want as a friend, being on the bus with someone who talks too much, breaking up with someone, avoiding starting a conversation in a store) and try using STOP skills effectively.

3. Situation 1 was: _____

   Describe how you used STOP skills in Situation 1 and your observations here.

4. Situation 2 was: _____

   Describe how you used STOP skills in Situation 2 and your observations here.

Time Management

Week	Date	Topic	Assignments (due the following week)
1		Assessment of Time versus Values and Ambitions	• Make estimates of how you spend your time. • Track your time. • Observe your values and ambitions, and how they relate to your time.
2		Developing an Ideal Time Map	• Develop an ideal time map that fits values and ambitions. • Track your time. • Observe and describe what you learn.
3		Developing a Trial Time Map	• Develop a trial time map. • Track your time. • Observe and describe what you learn.
4		Moving from the Trial Time Map to Your Schedule	• Revise your trial time map. • Track your time. • Make an effective schedule. • Observe and describe what you learn.

This module was adapted from *Time Management from the Inside Out* by Julie Morgenstern (2004). You may want to read or review the book as you participate in this module or watch online videos on this topic that Morgenstern has produced.

Week 1: Assessment of Time versus Values and Ambitions

This module is about time management—how you mindfully or mindlessly allocate the fixed 16 awake hours a day, which is 112 hours/week, or 5,840 hours/year.

112 hours	Let's start doing some math and estimate how your time is spent <u>now</u>:

So, how are you dividing up your 112 hours?

112 hours

Let's start doing some math and estimate how your time is spent <u>now</u>:

Work = _____ hrs/wk

School (class + studying) = _____ hrs/wk

Commuting = _____ hrs/wk

Appointments and errands = _____ hrs/wk

Cooking, cleaning, laundry, etc. = _____ hrs/wk

Partner/family = _____ hrs/wk

Friends/social = _____ hrs/wk

0 hours

56 hours

Clubs/activities = _____ hrs/wk

Exercise/fitness = _____ hrs/wk

Meditation = _____ hrs/wk

TV/video games = _____ hrs/wk

Social media = _____ hrs/wk

Other downtime/spare time = _____ hrs/wk

Sleep

_____ = _____ hrs/wk

_____ = _____ hrs/wk

_____ = _____ hrs/wk

0 hours   _____ = _____ hrs/wk

(continued)

Here is one completed example (of no one in particular, using one way of ordering activities):

Downtime 3
Reading 2
Social media 7
TV/video games 14
Exercise 4
Clubs/activities 2
Friends/social 5
Partner/family 10
Household 10
Appts/errands 5
Commuting 15
School 15
Work 20
Sleep *8 hrs/night*

112 hours

0 hours
56 hours

0 hours

Let's start doing some math and estimate how your time is spent <u>now</u>:

Work = <u>20</u> hrs/wk

School (class + studying) = <u>15</u> hrs/wk

Commuting = <u>15</u> hrs/wk

Appointments and errands = <u>5</u> hrs/wk

Cooking, cleaning, laundry, etc. = <u>10</u> hrs/wk

Partner/family = <u>10</u> hrs/wk

Friends/social = <u>5</u> hrs/wk

Clubs/activities = <u>2</u> hrs/wk

Exercise/fitness = <u>4</u> hrs/wk

Meditation = <u>0</u> hrs/wk

TV/video games = <u>14</u> hrs/wk

Social media = <u>7</u> hrs/wk

Other downtime/spare time = <u>3</u> hrs/wk

<u>Reading_____</u> = <u>2</u>___ hrs/wk

_____ = _____ hrs/wk

_____ = _____ hrs/wk

_____ = _____ hrs/wk

(continued)

In-Class Exercise

Let's try figuring out where you are <u>now</u>.

2. Divide up this box:

Sleep

112 hours

0 hours
56 hours

0 hours

1. Do your best to figure out what amount of time you are spending on what, *on average*:

Work = _____ hrs/wk

School (class + studying) = _____ hrs/wk

Commuting = _____ hrs/wk

Appointments and errands = _____ hrs/wk

Cooking, cleaning, laundry, etc. = _____ hrs/wk

Partner/family = _____ hrs/wk

Friends/social = _____ hrs/wk

Clubs/activities = _____ hrs/wk

Exercise/fitness = _____ hrs/wk

Meditation = _____ hrs/wk

TV/video games = _____ hrs/wk

Social media = _____ hrs/wk

Other downtime/spare time = _____ hrs/wk

_____ = _____ hrs/wk

_____ = _____ hrs/wk

_____ = _____ hrs/wk

_____ = _____ hrs/wk

Week 1 Assignment:
Assessment of Time versus Values and Ambitions

1. Mindfully and carefully, redo and revise your in-class estimates to best estimate how you spend your time. Practice nonjudgmental skills.

1b. Divide up this box:

112 hours

1a. Do your best to figure out what amount of time you are spending on what, *on average*:

Work = _____ hrs/wk

School (class + studying) = _____ hrs/wk

Commuting = _____ hrs/wk

Appointments and errands = _____ hrs/wk

Cooking, cleaning, laundry, etc. = _____ hrs/wk

Partner/family = _____ hrs/wk

Friends/social = _____ hrs/wk

0 hours

56 hours

Clubs/activities = _____ hrs/wk

Exercise/fitness = _____ hrs/wk

Meditation = _____ hrs/wk

TV/video games = _____ hrs/wk

Social media = _____ hrs/wk

Sleep

Other downtime/spare time = _____ hrs/wk

_____ = _____ hrs/wk

_____ = _____ hrs/wk

_____ = _____ hrs/wk

0 hours

_____ = _____ hrs/wk

(continued)

2. Start tracking how you spend your time. We have made our estimates, but nothing replaces getting real-time data.

    2a. This is easiest using an app such as Hours or Daylio for the iPhone or Jiffy, or a TimeLogger for Android. Given that apps change a lot, search your app store for "time tracking" to find an app that will work for you. If you want to go old-school, use the simple Activity Log chart (pp. 83–84).

    2b. Track your time to the best of your ability this week (and throughout this module). Bring a summary to group next week for discussion.

3. Let go of time and how you manage it for this next step. Go back to your ambition and values.

    3a. Review your ambition—copy it here:

    3b. Review your key values. Write them down here. (For help, you can review Standard DBT Emotion Regulation Handout 18: Values and Priorities List or Emotion Regulation Worksheet 11A: Getting from Values to Action Steps; Linehan, 2015.)

(continued)

4. Mindfully, nonjudgmentally, and effectively compare your time bar from Question 1, and your time tracking/Activity Log from Question 2, with your values and ambitions from Question 3.

   4a. Observations about where my current time management reflects my ambition? Where does it not reflect my ambition?

   4b. Observations about where my current time management reflects my key values? Where does it not reflect my key values?

Activity Log

Week of _____

TIME	Monday	Tuesday	Wednesday	Thursday	Friday	Saturday	Sunday
6:00 A.M.							
6:30							
7:00							
7:30							
8:00							
8:30							
9:00							
9:30							
10:00							
10:30							
11:00							
11:30							
Noon							
12:30 P.M.							

(continued)

Activity Log *(page 2 of 2)*

TIME	Monday	Tuesday	Wednesday	Thursday	Friday	Saturday	Sunday
1:00							
1:30							
2:00							
2:30							
3:00							
3:30							
4:00							
4:30							
5:00							
5:30							
6:00							
7:00							
8:00							
9:00							
10:00							
11:00							
Midnight							

Week 2: Developing an Ideal Time Map

A time map is a general plan for your time that includes EVERYTHING:

- Work, school, vocational activities
- Social and recreational activities
- Household responsibilities
- Health behaviors including shopping, cooking, exercise, sleeping
- Spiritual activities, mindfulness
- Downtime, spare time, unscheduled time
- Other:

A time map is NOT a schedule. You can't organize your day based on your time map as day-to-day life is too complicated and changeable.

Just as you start with a map when you are planning a trip, the map is not your only tool. On the road, you consider traffic and where you might want to take a detour, when you want to stop for the night, and whether to stop because you come upon a fascinating UFO, toilet, mini-bottle, or gelato museum (there actually are such museums). Making the trip without the map would be chaotic and perhaps frustrating. Making the trip only based on the map would be rigid and boring. Time maps are like that.

A time map can be as simple as the time bar we worked on last week. Or as complicated and detailed as examples you can find on the internet. Or anywhere in between. There's an example of a time map included in Appendix 5.

Ideal Time Map Goals:

- Assist you to match time to your values and ambitions.
- Assist you to recognize that time is like a closet—it is a fixed space in which everything has to fit—and help you to struggle with what to keep and what to toss, and how to organize what space you have for what you want.
- Assist you to ask yourself the hard questions about what time means for you, what you most care about.

(continued)

We'll start with an ideal time map. Think of this as a fresh start. Do not become distracted by practicalities or hopeless thoughts. It is important to be effective (not find the truth). Make a time map *as if* you have the skills you need to do it.

Worry thoughts you are having	Check the facts and opposite action

Week 2 Assignment: Ideal Time Map

1. Continue tracking how you spend your time using an app or the Activity Log provided on pp. 89–90.

2. Make an ideal time map. Use any format you want. A paper option that includes all the hours of the week is provided (pp. 91–92), but it might be easier to use a calendar app on the computer or draw a time bar on a blank sheet of paper. Or make a collage.

   Your goal is to create a map of how you would spend your time in an ideal world that would predictably lead you to achieve your ambition and values.

   Bring a copy to group to discuss.

   Make some observations at the end of the week:

3. Anything you learned or that surprised you about how your time was actually spent this week?

(continued)

4. Observations about the process of making the ideal time map:

5. Observations on how perfectionism or hopeless, helpless, or other worry thoughts interfered with your ability to make an ideal time map (if they did):

Activity Log

Week of _____

TIME	Monday	Tuesday	Wednesday	Thursday	Friday	Saturday	Sunday
6:00 A.M.							
6:30							
7:00							
7:30							
8:00							
8:30							
9:00							
9:30							
10:00							
10:30							
11:00							
11:30							
Noon							
12:30 P.M.							

(continued)

Activity Log *(page 2 of 2)*

TIME	Monday	Tuesday	Wednesday	Thursday	Friday	Saturday	Sunday
1:00							
1:30							
2:00							
2:30							
3:00							
3:30							
4:00							
4:30							
5:00							
5:30							
6:00							
7:00							
8:00							
9:00							
10:00							
11:00							
Midnight							

Ideal Time Map That Fits My Values and Ambition

TIME	Monday	Tuesday	Wednesday	Thursday	Friday	Saturday	Sunday
6:00 A.M.							
6:30							
7:00							
7:30							
8:00							
8:30							
9:00							
9:30							
10:00							
10:30							
11:00							
11:30							
Noon							
12:30 P.M.							

(continued)

91

Ideal Time Map That Fits My Values and Ambition *(page 2 of 2)*

TIME	Monday	Tuesday	Wednesday	Thursday	Friday	Saturday	Sunday
1:00							
1:30							
2:00							
2:30							
3:00							
3:30							
4:00							
4:30							
5:00							
5:30							
6:00							
7:00							
8:00							
9:00							
10:00							
11:00							
Midnight							

Week 3: Moving from the Ideal Time Map to a Trial Time Map

Now that you have an initial idea of how your week ACTUALLY goes and how you would like it to go in an IDEAL world, it is time to find a synthesis.

What activities are you already doing and might want to include on your trial time map?

What aspects of your ideal time map seem really unlikely to be pulled off in the near future, and your Wise Mind says to set aside for now?

What seems really important and worth the struggle to fit into your ideal time map?

(continued)

Which of these important things does your Wise Mind think should be included in the trial time map right away?

What skills and effective strategies can you apply to this process so worry thoughts, dysregulated emotions, or avoidance do not interfere?

Week 3 Assignment: Trial Time Map

1. Continue tracking how you spend your time using an app or the Activity Log provided (pp. 97–98).

2. Make a trial time map.* As with the ideal time map, use any format you want. A grid is provided, if helpful (pp. 99–100). It is fine to change the format if the previous one didn't work, or you got a better idea from someone else or the group discussion.

   Your goal is to develop a time map you can use as your big picture of time management over the next few months, one that balances feasibility with your ambition and values. (This is not your schedule, so don't put specific events on it—just a general map for an arbitrary week. Schedules will come into the picture next week.)

   Bring a copy to group to discuss.

   Make some observations at the end of the week:

3. Anything you learned or that surprised you about how your time was actually spent?

(continued)

*Time maps are adapted from the book *Time Management from the Inside Out* by Julie Morgenstern (2004). Published by Holt Press. Reprinted by permission.

4. Observations on the process of revising an ideal to a trial time map:

5. What skills or strategies did you use to manage perfectionism, hopeless, helpless, or other worry thoughts that arose (if they did)?

Activity Log

Week of _____

TIME	Monday	Tuesday	Wednesday	Thursday	Friday	Saturday	Sunday
6:00 A.M.							
6:30							
7:00							
7:30							
8:00							
8:30							
9:00							
9:30							
10:00							
10:30							
11:00							
11:30							
Noon							
12:30 P.M.							

(continued)

97

Activity Log *(page 2 of 2)*

TIME	Monday	Tuesday	Wednesday	Thursday	Friday	Saturday	Sunday
1:00							
1:30							
2:00							
2:30							
3:00							
3:30							
4:00							
4:30							
5:00							
5:30							
6:00							
7:00							
8:00							
9:00							
10:00							
11:00							
Midnight							

Trial Time Map That Balances Feasibility with My Values and Ambition

TIME	Monday	Tuesday	Wednesday	Thursday	Friday	Saturday	Sunday
6:00 A.M.							
6:30							
7:00							
7:30							
8:00							
8:30							
9:00							
9:30							
10:00							
10:30							
11:00							
11:30							
Noon							
12:30 P.M.							

(continued)

99

Trial Time Map That Balances Feasibility with My Values and Ambition *(page 2 of 2)*

TIME	Monday	Tuesday	Wednesday	Thursday	Friday	Saturday	Sunday
1:00							
1:30							
2:00							
2:30							
3:00							
3:30							
4:00							
4:30							
5:00							
5:30							
6:00							
7:00							
8:00							
9:00							
10:00							
11:00							
Midnight							

Week 4: Moving from the Trial Time Map to Your Schedule

Now that you have a better idea of how your time is spent and the big picture of your time from your time map, let's figure out how to get from a time map to an effective weekly schedule.

Time Management Guidelines for Scheduling:

1. Have one and only one calendar that you can get to when you need it.

2. Schedule your day realistically—with some padding for unexpected interruptions or tasks.

3. Schedule your to-do tasks on your calendar using your best estimates of time. If you can't complete something, reschedule it for another time.

4. Schedule breaks, stillness, relaxation, and recharging into your calendar as well as allowing for sufficient sleep and regular meals/snacks. Your goal is sustainability, and those with emotional disorders need more of this rejuvenation. If you have trouble with focus, schedule frequent breaks to exercise, stretch, or move around.

5. Schedule time to plan the day in the morning or at the end of the day for tomorrow. Things will change, and a cue and time are needed to regroup.

6. Check your schedule at least 3 times/day at routine times. Use reminders.

7. Question yourself regularly. Is the big picture of how I want to spend my time (i.e., my time map) reflected in my schedule? Not every week but most weeks?

8. Use a time-tracking app or Activity Log to check this periodically going forward.

Effectively Scheduling To-Do Tasks:

1. Batch, Balance, and Backbone

   - <u>Batch</u>: Put like tasks together and do them in a block.

   - <u>Batch</u>: Schedule task blocks for a duration that fits for you. One technique is to work in a "Pomodoro," meaning take a 5-minute break after a 25-minute block. Take a longer break after four Pomodoros. However, for some people, longer periods lead to more focus.

   - <u>Batch</u>: If you concentrate better in the evening, do more focused batches of tasks then and take care of email or routine tasks, in batches, earlier in the day.

   - <u>Batch</u>: Practice one-mindfully during a batch, shut the door or put up a sign, turn off beeps, close email, put your phone in a drawer, etc.

   - <u>Balance</u>: If you make yourself unavailable for too long, you will be interrupted. Give space for interruptions in your schedule between batches.

   - <u>Backbone</u>: Say no to distractions (phone, email, social media) until a break.

   - <u>Backbone</u>: Say no to other people when they interrupt you and tell them when you will get back to them or when they can check back.

(continued)

2. Do the most important two to three things first, so if derailed, key tasks still get done.

3. Don't start a new task until you finish or reschedule the one you're working on. Be one-mindful and practice skills to prevent avoidance. Move on only in Wise Mind.

4. Trouble starting? Set a 15-minute timer. When it goes off, reset if you are starting to focus. If it just isn't working, stop and reschedule the task.

5. Mindfully consider when to-do lists aren't getting done—too many tasks, too big tasks, getting distracted, avoiding? Problem-solve and try again.

Week 4 Assignment:
Moving from the Trial Time Map to Your Schedule

1. Continue tracking how you spend your time using an app or the Activity Log provided for 1 more week.

2. If needed, revise your trial time map based on what you learned last week and in today's discussion. Plan to use this one for a few months; see how it goes.

3. Now, let's take a look at your schedule and to-do list. Revise both based on the time management strategies from today's teaching plus the big picture of your time map. Select one calendar tool for your schedule and put *everything* there, rather than leaving information spread across multiple places. Balance effort and ease.

   Note which ideas you used to make your most effective schedule/to-do list:

4. Use your revised schedule and to-do list, and the principles taught this week to manage your time.

   Make some observations at the end of the week:

(continued)

5. Anything you learned or that surprised you about how your time was actually spent compared to your schedule?

6. Observations about the process of revising your schedule/to-dos to be more effective:

7. What skills or strategies did you apply to manage perfectionism, hopeless, helpless, or other worry thoughts that arose when making or using your schedule?

Activity Log

Week of _____

TIME	Monday	Tuesday	Wednesday	Thursday	Friday	Saturday	Sunday
6:00 A.M.							
6:30							
7:00							
7:30							
8:00							
8:30							
9:00							
9:30							
10:00							
10:30							
11:00							
11:30							
Noon							
12:30 P.M.							

(continued)

Activity Log (page 2 of 2)

TIME	Monday	Tuesday	Wednesday	Thursday	Friday	Saturday	Sunday
1:00							
1:30							
2:00							
2:30							
3:00							
3:30							
4:00							
4:30							
5:00							
5:30							
6:00							
7:00							
8:00							
9:00							
10:00							
11:00							
Midnight							

Revised Trial Time Map That Balances Feasibility with My Values and Ambition

TIME	Monday	Tuesday	Wednesday	Thursday	Friday	Saturday	Sunday
6:00 A.M.							
6:30							
7:00							
7:30							
8:00							
8:30							
9:00							
9:30							
10:00							
10:30							
11:00							
11:30							
Noon							
12:30 P.M.							

Revised Trial Time Map That Balances Feasibility with My Values and Ambition *(page 2 of 2)*

TIME	Monday	Tuesday	Wednesday	Thursday	Friday	Saturday	Sunday
1:00							
1:30							
2:00							
2:30							
3:00							
3:30							
4:00							
4:30							
5:00							
5:30							
6:00							
7:00							
8:00							
9:00							
10:00							
11:00							
Midnight							

Managing Emotions Effectively

Week	Date	Topic	Assignments (due the following week)
1		Assessment of Reducing Vulnerability Skills: What's Working and What's Not, and How to Change It	1. Do self-assessment of current skill practice. 2. Track Emotion Vulnerability skills on calendar charts, an app, or calendar. 3. Emotion Vulnerability Check-In.
2		Regulating Your Emotions When You Need to	1. Evaluate emotion dysregulation problems in three contexts. 2. Interview therapist about emotion dysregulation problems in each context.* 3. Develop and try an emotion regulation plan for each context.
3		Identifying and Managing Irritability	1. Self-assess irritability. 2. Manage three irritants.
4		Managing Anxiety with the Body and the Mind	1. Practice Progressive Relaxation twice/day for 1 week. 2. Practice asking the four questions twice: once for a current anxiety and once for a serious anxiety. 3. Complete Recovery Goals Self-Assessment to see how you are doing.

*This assignment involves a discussion with your individual therapist. Let your individual therapist know about the assignment at the beginning of session or ahead of time so you have time to discuss.

Week 1: Assessment of Reducing Vulnerability Skills:
What's Working and What's Not, and How to Change It

Skill	What parts/examples of this skill did you do before DBT?	What parts/ examples are you doing now?	Effective strategies that help me do this skill	Avoidance behaviors that block this skill
Treat Physical Illness				
Balanced Eating				
Avoid Mood-Altering Substances				
Balanced Sleep				
Balanced Exercise				

(continued)

From *DBT Next Steps Skills Handouts: Building a Life Worth Living*, by Katherine Anne Comtois, Adam Carmel, and Marsha M. Linehan. Copyright © 2025 The Guilford Press. Permission to photocopy this material or download it from the epdf is granted to purchasers of this book for personal use or use with clients; see copyright page for details.

What's Working and What's Not, and How to Change It *(page 2 of 4)*

Skill	What parts/examples of this skill did you do before DBT?	What parts/ examples are you doing now?	Effective strategies that help me do this skill	Avoidance behaviors that block this skill
Build Mastery				
Do a Positive a Day				
Work toward Long-Term Positives				
Attend to Relationships				
Cope Ahead of Time				

(continued)

112

So how do you improve your Reducing Vulnerability skills?

- This is a very difficult task for most people.
- These are the hardest skills to maintain long term, and there is a whole field of health psychology (not to mention life coaches, personal trainers, etc.) where professions are based on how difficult this is to maintain.
- In DBT Next Steps, we achieve in the face of difficulty using the Check-In.

Let's work through an example:

A Reducing Vulnerability <u>skill</u> I could practice more effectively (*Note:* Same guidelines apply as picking an Action Step for Check-In):

A <u>goal</u> that practicing this Reducing Vulnerability skill would help me achieve (like ambition, but think of specifically *how to achieve emotional invulnerability*):

(continued)

What are <u>effective</u> things I could do to practice my Reducing Vulnerability skill this week? (*Note:* Describe HOW you could get yourself to do the skill)

What are ways I could <u>avoid</u> practicing my Reducing Vulnerability skill this week? (*Note:* Describe what could block the skill, i.e., thoughts, decisions, or actions)

How could I apply the effective strategies to prevent avoidance?

Week 1 Assignment:
Assessment of Reducing Vulnerability Skills:
What's Working and What's Not, and How to Change It

1. Complete self-assessment from class thoroughly.

2. Track your current use of Reducing Vulnerability skills every day (you can use the handout provided on pp. 117–118, an app, or your calendar).

   For each day, note <u>when</u> you did the following things (and <u>how long</u>, if applicable):

   - Accumulate Positives:
     - Contact with others
     - Positives you prompted
     - Steps you took toward long-term positives
   - Build Mastery:
     - Activities that were challenging but possible
     - Activities you had been putting off or avoiding that you did or started on
   - Physical Illness:
     - When you took medications, vitamins, etc.
     - When you did recommended activities for physical health like physical therapy
   - Eating: <u>When</u> you ate (ignore *what* you ate for this exercise)
   - Mood-altering substances including caffeine and nicotine: when and what you used
   - Sleep:
     - When you got up
     - When you got into bed
     - When you fell asleep
     - Naps (if any)
   - Exercise: When, what, and how long

3. Complete Reducing Vulnerability Check-In to improve one Reducing Vulnerability skill of your choice.

   This week's Reducing Vulnerability <u>skill</u> (*Note:* Same guidelines apply as picking an Action Step for Check-In):

(continued)

<u>Goal</u> (how I can become emotionally invulnerable by practicing this Reducing Vulnerability skill, like ambition for Check-In):

*<u>Progress</u> (*Note:* Present the part you achieved first and then the part you did not achieve, if any, i.e., avoid judgment):

One <u>effective</u> thing I did to practice my Reducing Vulnerability skill this week (*Note:* Describe HOW you got yourself to do the skill; don't just restate your progress):

One way I <u>avoided</u> practicing my Reducing Vulnerability skill this week, if I did. (*Note:* Describe what blocked using the skill, i.e., thoughts, decisions, or actions):

**If I avoided, one way I will <u>prevent this avoidance</u> behavior in the future is (*Note:* Give a skills or strategy like those in the effective behavior section):

---

*Group focus is on giving positive reinforcement.

**Group focus is on problem solving and goal setting when needed, because coaching others teaches yourself as well.

Reducing Vulnerability Skill Tracking Calendar

TIME	Monday	Tuesday	Wednesday	Thursday	Friday	Saturday	Sunday
6:00 A.M.							
6:30							
7:00							
7:30							
8:00							
8:30							
9:00							
9:30							
10:00							
10:30							
11:00							
11:30							
Noon							
12:30 P.M.							

(continued)

117

Reducing Vulnerability Skill Tracking Calendar *(page 2 of 2)*

TIME	Monday	Tuesday	Wednesday	Thursday	Friday	Saturday	Sunday
1:00							
1:30							
2:00							
2:30							
3:00							
3:30							
4:00							
4:30							
5:00							
5:30							
6:00							
7:00							
8:00							
9:00							
10:00							
11:00							
Midnight							

118

Week 2: Regulating Yourself When You Need It

Let's discuss where the most important problem areas are for you as you move forward into a stable life off disability connected to a community you love who loves you.

Consider which of these situations are a problem because of your emotion dysregulation (or by numbing out, dissociating, or some other response to dysregulation).

Check off the problems you have associated with emotion dysregulation.

Work or School Context

- ☐ With my supervisor
- ☐ My office mate
- ☐ Being bored
- ☐ Staying too late
- ☐ Obsessing
- ☐ No feedback
- ☐ Following directions
- ☐ _____
- ☐ _____

- ☐ With criticism
- ☐ Staff meetings
- ☐ Being on time
- ☐ Taking extra shifts
- ☐ Being physically ill
- ☐ Invalidating feedback
- ☐ Doing too little
- ☐ _____
- ☐ _____

- ☐ Wondering what others think
- ☐ Performance evaluations
- ☐ Getting to work
- ☐ Checking out
- ☐ Not completing homework
- ☐ Undoing positive feedback
- ☐ Doing too much
- ☐ _____

Social Context

- ☐ With my family
- ☐ During a fight
- ☐ Being bored
- ☐ Avoiding new people
- ☐ Judging others
- ☐ Meeting new people
- ☐ Texting too much
- ☐ Maintaining contact
- ☐ Being criticized
- ☐ _____
- ☐ _____

- ☐ With my friends
- ☐ Being ignored
- ☐ Feeling disconnected
- ☐ Stuck on being right
- ☐ Lack of patience
- ☐ Reconnecting
- ☐ Overchecking texts
- ☐ Being lonely
- ☐ Asking for help
- ☐ _____
- ☐ _____

- ☐ With my partner
- ☐ Ending relationships
- ☐ Keeping constant GIVE
- ☐ Feeling taken advantage of
- ☐ Feeling taken for granted
- ☐ Managing social media
- ☐ Responding in Emotion Mind
- ☐ Keeping constant FAST
- ☐ Backing off when needed
- ☐ _____

(continued)

Self-Management Context

- ☐ Impulsive purchases
- ☐ Paying down debt
- ☐ Overbooked
- ☐ Too much alone time
- ☐ Overcommitting
- ☐ Managing illness
- ☐ Planning for depression
- ☐ _____
- ☐ _____

- ☐ Staying within budget
- ☐ Dealing with creditors
- ☐ Too little downtime
- ☐ Not enough alone time
- ☐ People pleasing
- ☐ Managing pain
- ☐ Keeping to a routine
- ☐ _____
- ☐ _____

- ☐ Making a budget
- ☐ Avoiding money issues
- ☐ Too much downtime
- ☐ Emotion Mind time management
- ☐ Not observing own limits
- ☐ Managing doctors
- ☐ Sleep–wake cycle
- ☐ _____

Remember how to regulate your emotions when you need to:

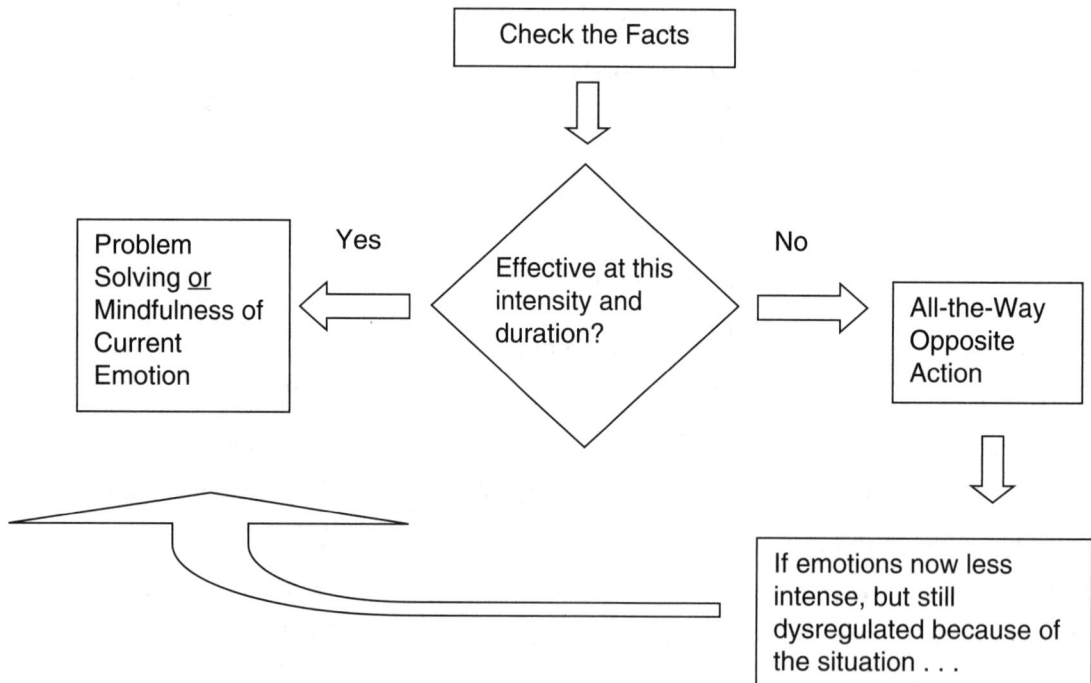

```
                    Check the Facts
                          |
                          v
Problem Solving or    Effective at this       All-the-Way
Mindfulness of  <-Yes- intensity and  -No->   Opposite
Current Emotion        duration?              Action
                                                 |
                                                 v
                                      If emotions now less
                                      intense, but still
                                      dysregulated because of
                                      the situation . . .
```

(continued)

Let's work through an example:

1. Describe a work, social, or self-management context that creates a problem due to your emotional dysregulation:

2. What is the dominant emotion? _____

3. Check the Facts. If not, redescribe. Decide if emotion is justified and effective.

4. Based on the flowchart above, decide your emotion solution.

If effective, Problem-Solve or use Mindfulness of Current Emotion. If not, figure out *All-the-Way Opposite Action*.

Week 2 Assignment: Regulating Yourself When You Need It

1. Conduct an individual assessment of yourself to figure out key contexts that are emotion dysregulation problems for you.

2. Interview your therapist to identify key contexts that they have observed dysregulating you. Be curious.

Top Work or School Contexts That Dysregulate Me

I identify:

1.

2.

3.

4.

5.

My therapist identifies (may be the same or a different list):

1.

2.

3.

4.

5.

Top Social Contexts That Dysregulate Me

I identify:

1.

2.

3.

(continued)

4.

5.

My therapist identifies (may be the same or a different list):

1.

2.

3.

4.

5.

Top Self-Management Contexts That Dysregulate Me

I identify:

1.

2.

3.

4.

5.

My therapist identifies (may be the same or a different list):

1.

2.

3.

4.

5.

Practice figuring out an emotion regulation plan for your top work/school, social, and self-management contexts. *(You may want to divide the week into three 2- to 3-day periods and work on one plan in each.)*

(continued)

Top <u>Work or School</u> Context

1. Describe a *work or school context* that creates a problem due to your emotional dysregulation:

2. What is the dominant emotion? _____

3. Check the Facts. If not, redescribe. Decide if emotion is justified and effective.

4. Based on the flowchart above, decide your emotion solution. If effective, Problem-Solve or use Mindfulness of Current Emotion. If not, figure out *All-the-Way* Opposite Action.

5. If context arises (or you could make it arise) this week, do the plan. Observe and describe the results. Where could you tweak the plan to make it more effective?

(continued)

Top <u>Social</u> Context

1. Describe a *social context* that creates a problem due to your emotional dysregulation:

2. What is the dominant emotion? _____

3. Check the Facts. If not, redescribe. Decide if emotion is justified and effective.

4. Based on the flowchart above, decide your emotion solution. If effective, Problem-Solve or use Mindfulness of Current Emotion. If not, figure out *All-the-Way* Opposite Action.

5. If context arises (or you could make it arise) this week, do the plan. Observe and describe the results. Where could you tweak the plan to make it more effective?

(continued)

Top <u>Self-Management</u> Context

1. Describe a *self-management context* that creates a problem due to your emotional dysregulation:

2. What is the dominant emotion? _____

3. Check the Facts. If not, redescribe. Decide if emotion is justified and effective.

4. Based on the flowchart above, decide your emotion solution. If effective, Problem-Solve or use Mindfulness of Current Emotion. If not, figure out *All-the-Way* Opposite Action.

5. If context arises (or you could make it arise) this week, do the plan. Observe and describe the results. Where could you tweak the plan to make it more effective?

Week 3: Identifying and Managing Irritability

To manage irritability, it is first critical to identify that irritability (or its relations "aggravation," "frustration," or "exasperation") is present:

- When/where/how do you experience irritability or its relations?
- When/where do others say you are irritable? Who says this?
- When/where/how do you make judgments, think shoulds (including "hidden" shoulds), or make assumptions or generalizations about how the world is or should be?
- When/where/how are others (who?) withdrawing from you, decreasing eye contact, giving in, pacifying, patronizing, or otherwise responding to you as if to an angry or irritable person?

Notes and examples:

(continued)

What is irritability?

Merriam-Webster's dictionary defines it as:

1. the quality or state of being irritable; readiness to become annoyed or angry
2. the property of living tissue and living things that permits them to react to stimuli

Other terms are "cross," "petulant," "cantankerous," "bad-tempered," "prickly," "tetchy," "irascible," "touchy," "testy," "grouchy."

Experiences (sensing) of irritability might include:

- Nerve endings agitated
- Malaise
- Oversensitivity
- Inconsolability

What makes irritability different from anger?

Irritants (i.e., prompting events or vulnerability factors):

- Tired
- Overloaded
- Outside of personal limits
- Lack of downtime
- Hormonal changes
- Lack of nutrition
- Dehydration

(continued)

- Imbalance of wants to shoulds
- Low blood sugar
- Being around critical people (including yourself)
- Being around invalidating people (including yourself)
- Being ignored or taken for granted (including by yourself)
- Being around another person's negative emotions
- Feeling alone or lonely

Which of these irritants apply to you, where, and how?

Irritability = Irritants/Aversive sensations + Thoughts that it shouldn't be like this

Thoughts that exacerbate irritability:
- Shouldn't be this way
- "Can't" thoughts ("can't take this," "can't stand this," "can't go on like this," . . .)
- Hopeless
- Helpless
- Defeated
- Victimized
- Unfair
- Personalizing
- Threatened
- Catastrophizing or "awful-izing"

(continued)

Only five possible responses to irritability:

1. Remove irritant:

   - If hungry, eat.
   - If tired, balance sleep or take a mini-vacation.
   - If overloaded, figure out and follow time management strategy.

2. Change how you feel about the irritant:

   - If hungry, recognize that it makes sense and is temporary.
   - If tired, act opposite to the irritability and participate positively.
   - If overloaded, be grateful for the opportunities that are taking your time.

3. Accept and tolerate the irritant:

   - If hungry, distract and transfer your attention to something else.
   - If tired, self-soothe with the scent of lavender, takeout, a good movie.
   - If overloaded, radically accept that you have made choices and half-smile.

4. Stay miserable:

   - If hungry, don't find a way to get a meal or snack in.
   - If tired, just keep going and tell yourself you should be able to do it.
   - If overloaded, think of yourself as a victim who is stuck with the tasks you've got.

5. Make it worse:

   - If hungry, act impatiently with those around you.
   - If tired, be mad at yourself for acting irritable or being so tired.
   - If overloaded, blame others for asking so much of you.

Thus, reducing irritability requires choosing one or more of the first three options:

1. *Change the situation* by reducing or getting rid of the irritant.
2. *Change how you feel or think about the situation* to make it less irritating.
3. *Radically accept and tolerate the irritant,* turning the mind toward accepting the irritant, and have a willingness to do what is needed to tolerate the irritant without making things worse.

How does this apply to you?

Week 3 Assignment: Identifying and Managing Irritability

1. For each day, give a rating of average/highest anger and irritability. Then, check off which aspects of anger or irritability occurred on that day (i.e., in any of the situations where you felt angry or irritable).

	Thurs	Fri	Sat	Sun	Mon	Tues	Wed
Average anger for the day/highest anger (0–5/0–5)	/	/	/	/	/	/	/
Average irritation for the day/highest irritation (0–5/0–5)	/	/	/	/	/	/	/
Breathing changes							
Muscle tension							
Angry or irritable body posture							
Thinking things aren't the way you want them to be or what you want is being blocked							
Judgmental thoughts, assumptions, or interpretations you can't support with observable facts							
Said judgmental, irritable, or angry words							
Nonjudgmental in words, but angry or irritable thoughts							
Someone verbally observed you were angry							
Someone verbally observed you were irritable							
Someone withdrew physically							
Someone stopped or avoided eye contact							
Someone gave in on something they likely didn't want to							
Someone patronized you or was condescending toward you							
Something else that told you they found you to be angry							

(continued)

131

2. What are your 10 top irritants?

1.	2.
3.	4.
5.	6.
7.	8.
9.	10.

How have you stayed miserable or made your misery worse in the face of these irritants?

3. For your top three irritants, describe how you <u>could</u> use the more effective options:

Irritant 1: _____

Remove irritant by:

Change how you feel about the irritant by:

Accept/tolerate the irritant by:

Practice using one or more of these effective options this week.

Observe and Describe your experience of the irritant and how you handled it this week:

(continued)

Irritant 2: _____

Remove irritant by:

Change how you feel about the irritant by:

Accept/tolerate the irritant by:

Practice using one or more of these effective options this week.

Observe and Describe your experience of the irritant and how you handled it this week:

Irritant 3: _____

Remove irritant by:

Change how you feel about the irritant by:

Accept/tolerate the irritant by:

Practice using one or more of these effective options this week.

Observe and Describe your experience of the irritant and how you handled it this week:

Week 4: Managing Anxiety with the Body and the Mind

Progressive Muscle Relaxation for Anxiety Reduction through the Body

If you have an anxiety disorder, meaning that anxiety is interfering with your optimal functioning in a significant way, it is often the case that your body is in a fairly constant state of alertness and vigilance. While having a body on alert in this manner is helpful in an immediately dangerous environment, it is generally not helpful when the environment is not immediately threatening. Part of recognizing and reducing unhelpful anxiety can be learning first to become aware of tension held in the body and second to have the ability to release that tension. Relaxed muscles send a message to the brain that the environment is safe, making it easier for your mind to stop scanning for what might go wrong.

This module, Managing Anxiety with the Body and the Mind, will include twice-daily homework that will move you almost completely through the entire Progressive Muscle Relaxation (PMR) protocol (Barlow & Craske, 2007). The exercises in the protocol are designed to:

1. Increase your awareness of muscular tension.
2. Help you to release tension effectively and get to a relaxed state.
3. Notice earlier when muscular tension is starting to build in your body.
4. Increase your practice in concentrating your awareness (Mindfulness).
5. Associate the word "relax" with relaxed muscles so that ultimately you will be able to achieve a state of relaxation rapidly across contexts.

As you prepare to engage in practice, make sure that you have enough (as much as 30 minutes) of uninterrupted time. If possible, change into clothing that will not bind or interfere with your breath or comfort. You may choose to sit in a straight-backed chair or to lie down on the floor or your bed. If you find that you fall asleep during the exercise, choose a chair for the next practice. The goal is to achieve a relaxed state with awareness, not to fall asleep.

Longer practices (20–30 minutes) are better if you have difficulty with relaxation as they give more opportunity for relaxing each muscle before moving on. Over time, shorter options will become more effective as your body learns to relax.

Note: PMR instructions generally suggest that you will notice sensations of relaxation. It is possible that you will <u>not</u> at first experience the sensations described. It is important that you remind yourself that what you are practicing is observing sensations associated with the physical act of tensing muscles, contrasted with sensations of relaxing that tension. Try to let go of your ideas of what that should be. Practice observing whatever sensations are present nonjudgmentally, letting go of them

(continued)

as they arise. This process cannot be forced. It may take some time for your body to let go. Keep practicing.

16-Muscle-Group Procedure

Start first with each of the 16 muscle groups (Linehan, 2015).

Once you can do that, practice with medium groups of muscles and then large groups.

Once you are good at that, practice tensing your entire body at once.

When you tense your entire body, you are like a robot—stiff, nothing moving.

When you relax your entire body, you are like a rag doll—all muscles drooping down.

Once you can relax all your muscles, practice three or four times a day until you can routinely relax your entire body rapidly.

By practicing pairing exhaling and the word "relax" with relaxing your muscles, you will eventually be able to relax just by letting go and saying the word "relax."

Large Medium Small

1. Hands and wrists: Make fists with both hands and pull fists up on the wrists.
2. Lower and upper arms: Make fists and bend both arms up to touch your shoulders.
3. Shoulders: Pull both shoulders up to your ears.
4. Forehead: Pull eyebrows close together, wrinkling forehead.
5. Eyes: Shut eyes tightly.
6. Nose and upper cheeks: Scrunch up nose; bring upper lips and cheeks up toward eyes.
7. Lips and lower face: Press lips together; bring edges of lips back toward ears.
8. Tongue and mouth: Teeth together; tongue pushing on upper mouth.
9. Neck: Push head back into chair, floor, or bed, or push chin down to chest.
10. Chest: Take deep breath and hold it.
11. Back: Arch back, bringing shoulder blades together.
12. Stomach: Hold stomach in tightly.
13. Buttocks: Squeeze buttocks together.
14. Upper legs and thighs: Legs out; tense thighs.
15. Calves: Legs out; point toes down.
16. Ankles: Legs out; point toes together, heels out, toes curled under.

Apart from the 16-muscle-group procedure listed above (Linehan, 2015), there are many other PMR procedures available, including audio clips, apps, and additional written materials. You can listen to audio clips and follow along, or ask your individual therapist to make a recording for you to listen to and practice. The weekly assignments will clarify which of these procedures to use when (e.g., using a 16-muscle-group PMR procedure vs. an 8-muscle-group PMR procedure). Consider the following PMR resources:

- www.va.gov/WHOLEHEALTHLIBRARY/tools/progressive-muscle-relaxation.asp
- www.umcvc.org/health-library/uz2225+
- www.youtube.com/watch?v=ihO02wUzgkc

(continued)

135

Recall Relaxation Training Procedure

When PMR practice takes place for at least 3 weeks, you will likely be more conscious of how your muscles feel when tightened as compared to relaxed. If you have reached the ability to find a state of relaxation during the 4-muscle-group relaxation procedure and you're over 70 on the scale of relaxation below, you may want to stop the 16-muscle-group procedure in the evening and only practice the recall procedure we are about to describe. However, if you find that you are not yet reaching this level of relaxation with the 4-muscle-group procedure, you may want to continue with the 16-muscle-group procedure above once per day and the new recall procedure once per day.

PMR Scale of Relaxation

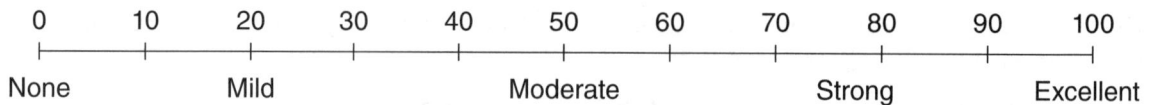

0	10	20	30	40	50	60	70	80	90	100
None		Mild			Moderate			Strong		Excellent

For the Recall Relaxation procedure, practice the following: Focus your mind on each of the four muscle groups sequentially for 20 seconds. While you are focusing your mind, remember the feelings of relaxation as experienced during your previous exercises. Imagine that you are experiencing them now. You may want to think of sensations of heaviness, warmth, floating, or any sensation or imagery helpful to you in reaching a relaxed state. You may also want to consciously let your physical body droop (e.g., the shoulders) or let go of any held tension in your jaw. Once you have moved your mind through all the muscle groups in this manner, focus on slow breathing for 1 to 2 minutes. Remember to say the word "relax" on the out breath to yourself for the whole time. Finally, count backward to 1 again to wake yourself out of a deep state of relaxation (Barlow & Craske, 2007).

Once you are able to successfully relax during the Recall Relaxation procedure, you are ready for the next step. You may not be completely relaxed, but there is a clear difference that you can observe and you feel noticeably more relaxed.

Cue-Controlled Relaxation Procedures

Right now, think of the word "relax," and as you think of it, review your body and let go of all the tension within at once. Practice this throughout your day, as often as you can, any time you have a few seconds. You may pick some reminders to practice so you don't forget, such as a gentle phone alarm, stoplights, phone ringing, or getting a text. Also, begin to apply cue relaxation when you notice physical tension or anxiety start to build. The goal is to practice a competing response to fight, flight, or freeze.

(continued)

Notes

Each person differs in the length of time it takes them to reach a state of relaxation with these procedures. Some people have had tension in their body for so long, the muscles have to essentially learn how to relax and it takes practice for them to reach that stage. Until then, there will be only small or subtle differences between the tensed and relaxed states, and close, mindful observation is required to notice them. Other people who have rarely been relaxed like this may notice unfamiliar sensations (like floating), which are startling or trigger anxiety and tension. Exposure to the sensations of relaxation with repeated practice will teach the mind that these sensations are not threatening and the body will stop tensing. Some people feel as if they are not properly on guard when they are relaxed. If this is the case, it is important to Check the Facts and remember that dangerous things in the world are not changed by whether or not your body is relaxed. Opposite Action to anxiety is often needed to practice PMR when anxious or otherwise emotionally dysregulated.

This is a skill that requires extensive practice for maximum results. Keep it up and you should experience significant improvement in your efforts to master the effects of anxiety on your life.

Discuss the pace of your PMR procedures with your individual therapist to determine if the pace set for the group is right for you. If your therapist thinks a slower pace would be more effective for you, come up with a plan to keep the process going in individual therapy so you reach the same endpoint (even if the group is moving on to the next module).

Four Questions to Manage Anxiety with Your Mind

Use your *Wise Mind* to answer the following questions about what you are afraid will happen in a situation of serious anxiety: _____

(Describe a current or past situation above.)

1. What is the WORST thing that can happen? (If more than one, do a sheet for each worst thing.)

2. How LIKELY (from 0 to 100%) is it the worst thing will occur? _____%

0%	50%	100%
Impossible it will occur		No doubt that it will occur

3. How BAD would the worst thing actually be? _____

0	5	10
Piece of cake		The truly <u>worst</u> thing you can imagine

4. What skills would you use, or how would you cope if the worst thing did occur? Make a list of skills and effective behaviors you would utilize. Stick with this until you have an effective plan.

Week 4 Assignment:
Managing Anxiety with the Body and the Mind

1. Practice Progressive Relaxation 16-muscle group twice a day. Move to 8-muscle relaxation if numbers get above 70 (based on the relaxation scale below).

   You can use any Progressive Relaxation tape, etc. that is at least 20 minutes or is explicitly divided into 16 muscle groups.

   You may not become relaxed at first if you are a very anxious person. It takes regular repetition for your muscles to let go and it may also feel weird at first.

PMR Scale of Relaxation

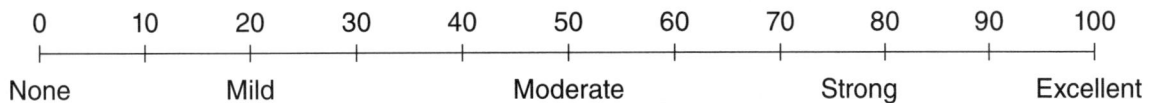

0	10	20	30	40	50	60	70	80	90	100
None		Mild			Moderate			Strong		Excellent

Date	Describe practice	Relaxation at the end of exercise	Concentration during the exercise

Consult with your individual therapist, as needed, to find a modified practice if Progressive Relaxation is too challenging for you.

2. Complete both versions of the Four Questions to Manage Anxiety with Your Thoughts worksheet: The first specifies a <u>current</u> fear or anxiety that arises this week (serious or mild), and the second concerns <u>serious</u> fear (past or present).

Four Questions to Manage Anxiety with Your Thoughts

Use your *Wise Mind* to answer the following questions about what you are afraid will happen in a situation of <u>current</u> anxiety: _____ (Describe a mild or serious situation.)

1. What is the WORST thing that can happen? (If more than one, do a sheet for each worst thing.)

2. How LIKELY (from 0 to 100%) is it the worst thing will occur? _____%

0%   50%   100%
├─────────────────────────────────────┼─────────────────────────────────────┤
Impossible it will occur   No doubt that it will occur

3. How BAD would the worst thing actually be? _____

0   5   10
├─────────────────────────────────────┼─────────────────────────────────────┤
Piece of cake   The truly <u>worst</u> thing
                                                                     you can imagine

4. What skills would you use, or how would you cope if the worst thing did occur? Make a list of skills and effective behaviors you would utilize. Stick with this until you have an effective plan.

Four Questions to Manage Anxiety with Your Thoughts

Use your *Wise Mind* to answer the following questions about what you are afraid will happen in a situation of <u>serious</u> anxiety: _____. (Describe a current, past, or future situation.)

1. What is the WORST thing that can happen? (If more than one, do a sheet for each worst thing.)

2. How LIKELY (from 0 to 100%) is it the worst thing will occur? _____%

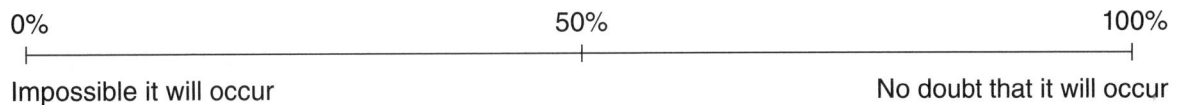

0%   50%   100%
├──────────────────────────────────┼──────────────────────────────────┤
Impossible it will occur   No doubt that it will occur

3. How BAD would the worst thing actually be? _____

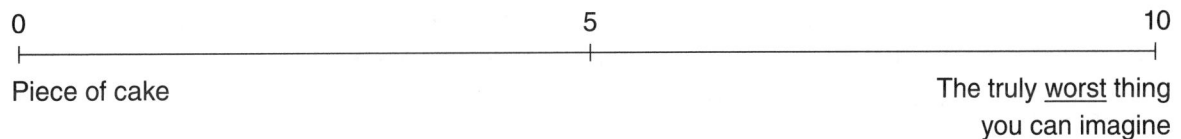

0   5   10
├──────────────────────────────────┼──────────────────────────────────┤
Piece of cake   The truly <u>worst</u> thing
                                                           you can imagine

4. What skills would you use, or how would you cope if the worst thing did occur? Make a list of skills and effective behaviors you would utilize. Stick with this until you have an effective plan.

Self-Assessment of DBT Next Steps Recovery Goals

Name:	Months into DBT Next Steps:	Date:

1. Please note how far you have come on each of these Recovery Goals that are the focus of DBT Next Steps on the following scale and check which Recovery Goals you are currently working on with your individual therapist.

0 = Not thought about it or talked about it

1 = Thought or talked about it, no action, don't want to

2 = Thought or talked about it, no action, want to

3 = Tried to do/get it but couldn't

4 = Trying to do it, can do/have it, once or twice

5 = Trying to do it, can do/have it, not reliably

6 = Do/have this reliably, still have problems being effective

7 = Do/have this reliably, this problem is essentially solved

Recovery Goals	Number	✓ if current target
Living Wage Employment and Off Psychiatric Disability		
Choose a career path to living wage employment knowing its fit with your Wise Mind values and talents as well as the practical issues of pay, health insurance, leave and retirement benefits, hours, shift times, required training or certification, and routes to advancement.		
Demonstrate capability to financially support yourself (and your family) in your chosen career without psychiatric disability payments or partner's/family's income.		
Demonstrate capability to financially support yourself (and your family) in at least one fallback job without psychiatric disability payments or partner's/family's income (if needed).		
Sufficient health insurance to maintain health care and medications.		
Better than 90% follow-through at work on attendance, being on time, appropriate dress and manner, following directions, and job tasks.		

(continued)

Recovery Goals	Number	✓ if current target
Interpersonal Proficiency		
Interpersonally easy to work/be with—even with difficult people and during stressful times.		
Demonstrate capability to regulate emotional expression and actions, and find Wise Mind in all interpersonal situations—even with difficult people and during stressful times.		
Know your Wise Mind personal limits and act on them with yourself, employer, friends, family, colleagues, and members of your community.		
Receive praise, raises, promotions, and offers for more desirable jobs and roles within your community.		
Life Outside Work *(Note: These categories are expected to overlap.)*		
Have at least a couple of local and/or long-distance friends whose values align with yours.		
Have at least one person or group for casual interactions (e.g., lunchroom, church, coffee, movie, book club, volunteer organization).		
Have at least one close support with whom you experience intimacy and discuss private issues (who is not your therapist).		
Have at least one local person or group that would notice you were not around and would take action to find you.		
Be an active member of an organized recreational activity that is either fun or meaningful and not related to mental health (e.g., volunteer organization, church, sports teams, Spanish lessons, ballroom dancing).		
Disengage from relationships with family members that are ineffective or destructive.		
Disengage or end friendships that are ineffective or destructive.		
Choose relationships based on evidence that they are compatible with your lifestyle, needs, and values.		
Take steps to find an effective and rewarding romantic relationship (if desired).		

(continued)

143

Recovery Goals	Number	✓ if current target
Emotional Proficiency		
Able to experience negative emotions building, staying, and falling mindfully—not avoiding, rushing them along, or mentally moving into a different moment.		
Able to experience positive emotions building, staying, and falling mindfully—not avoiding, rushing them along, or mentally moving into a different moment.		
Able to reduce problematic emotions effectively and fast enough to prevent them from leading to problems.		
Self-Management		
Have an effective method for managing your monthly budget and one-time expenses (e.g., new tires) so you stay within your income.		
Sufficient emergency fund savings to cover 3 months of living expenses in case you lose your job.		
Have an effective method of savings for things you would enjoy.		
Have an effective method for getting out of debt/getting debt to a reasonable level.		
Have an effective method for managing your time that means spending your time in line with your Wise Mind values.		
Have an effective method for managing your time that gets key things done on time.		
Have an effective method for managing your time that balances work, leisure, household, and downtime.		
Have an effective method of preventing illness and psychiatric symptoms from impacting your functioning.		
Have an effective method of managing chronic illness or pain to minimize its impact on your quality of life.		

(continued)

2. One of the characteristics of a life worth living outside of mental health is significant responsibilities that require time, timeliness, follow-through, patience, interest, creativity, etc. These responsibilities tend to benefit one's mental health. We'd like to know what responsibilities you have and whether they are something established that isn't requiring a lot of effort or something that you are starting to work on and requires significant attention.

	✓ the appropriate box	
List people, places, and things that I am responsible for/to:	**Established/ easy**	**Just starting/ challenging**

Succeeding after DBT

Week	Date	Topic	Assignments (due the following week)
1		Practicing DBT 24/7	Practice DBT 24/7.
2		Therapy-Interfering Behavior	Evaluate your remaining Therapy-Interfering Behaviors.*
3		Your Future and Therapy	Consider what treatment (if any) you want after completing DBT Next Steps.*
4		Practice Making Non-DBT Treatment Work	Role-play, twice, effective interactions with non-DBT providers.*

*This assignment involves a discussion with your individual therapist. Let your individual therapist know about the assignment at the beginning of session or ahead of time so you have time to discuss.

Week 1: Practice DBT 24/7

Ask yourself the following questions:

1. What percentage of the day are you acting effectively and using DBT skills? _____%

2. What percentage of the day do you think you need to be in Wise Mind and using DBT skills to fully achieve your 5-year ambitions? _____%

3. What percentage of the day do you need to consciously use DBT skills (rather than skills happening naturally and without effort)? _____%?

4. List situations/emotions/cues that interfere with being effective more often.

5. Circle your level of commitment, right now, to using skills to be effective 24/7?

   1   2   3   4   5   6   7   8   9   10

   None   Most important thing

6. Check whichever ideas below might increase your commitment. Consider adding new ideas, too.

   ☐ Imagining your life in 5 years with and without being effective?

   ☐ Having some sort of reminder (alarm, cheat sheet) to ask yourself in the moment, "Am I being effective?"

   ☐ Asking yourself in this moment, "Am I being willful?" If so, becoming willing.

   ☐ Reducing willfulness by asking, "What is the threat?" and "How can I deal with it?"

   ☐ List of sufficient distress tolerance skills to carry you through the worst moments.

   ☐ List of plans for both effectively distracting and for effectively accepting.

   ☐ Plan regular "vacations" or an "emergency break"—an escape that won't harm you.

   ☐ Borrowing someone else's faith, so you don't have to count on your own alone.

   ☐ Distract yourself in the moment from hopelessness and doubt—your doubts may be true, but they are your mortal enemy. (*Note:* Overly optimistic people tend to be very successful.)

Week 1 Assignment: Practice DBT 24/7

1. Choose at least three of the ideas in Question 6 (p. 149). Starting with them, develop a plan that is likely to increase your commitment to practicing DBT skills 24/7. Describe your plan here (use extra paper to describe the plan if needed).

2. Right after Question 1 above, circle your level of commitment to using skills to be effective 24/7.

    1   2   3   4   5   6   7   8   9   10

    None   Most important thing

3. Using your plan, practice *for 1 week* being effective every single minute (i.e., using DBT skills 24/7). This means jumping right back in whenever you fall off.

    Do this with the goal of observing the experience *for this week.* (We're not asking you do this in an ongoing way.)

4. At the end of the week, make some observations:

    a. What do you observe was hard or you didn't like about practicing DBT 24/7?

    b. What were the most valuable/helpful aspects of practicing DBT 24/7?

    c. What distress tolerance or acceptance skills were of the most help to pull off your practice?

5. Right before group, circle your level of commitment to using skills to be effective 24/7 as you go ahead.

    1   2   3   4   5   6   7   8   9   10

    None   Most important thing

Week 2: Therapy-Interfering Behaviors

1. Research and a century of clinical experience have shown that patients with problems with emotion regulation, interpersonal sensitivity, or distress tolerance fare badly in many traditional treatments including psychotherapy and community mental health. Possible reasons include:

   a. They tend to be more sensitive to therapeutic mistakes by their therapists.

   b. They tend to have more TIBs than other patients (more on this later).

   c. They do not benefit from medications as much as other folks. (There is no medication for emotion dysregulation per se.)

   d. They often get worse with case management as case management services tend to do things FOR you, rather than allowing you to do things for yourself.

   What problems have you had in mental health treatment?

   What has been more effective about your DBT treatment?

(continued)

2. Individuals with problems of emotion regulation, interpersonal sensitivity, or distress tolerance are exquisitely sensitive to their environment's response to them.

   Here is a list of some therapist behaviors that have interfered with individuals having effective therapy. **Which apply to you?**

   ☐ Unclear goals?

   ☐ Unclear time frame for treatment?

   ☐ Therapist insufficiently trained or skilled to solve your problems?

   ☐ Impatient or disrespectful behaviors?

   ☐ Becomes emotionally dysregulated in response to your behavior or statements?

   ☐ Doesn't know an effective treatment for your diagnosis and related problems?

   ☐ Reinforcing you for being sick (e.g., gave more help as symptoms escalated, reinforcing further escalation)?

   ☐ Failing to reinforce you for being effective (e.g., did not provide more help when you were working hard to solve or accept problems)?

   ☐ Acting like the treatment they are doing is more important than the relationship?

   ☐ Too soothing/validating/nurturing?

   ☐ Too demanding or change-focused?

   ☐ Not recognizing the efforts you did make?

   ☐ Being defensive about their mistakes?

   ☐ Emotionally dysregulated from fear of you being angry at them, suing them, or that you will commit suicide?

   ☐ Inability to tolerate how you are communicating your suffering in the moment?

   ☐ Trying to make it better in a way that reinforces your problem behaviors?

   ☐ Unrealistic beliefs of what is possible in the moment?

   ☐ "Fragilizing" you or expecting too little of you?

   ☐ Unwilling to accept you and your life—judgmental about your life choices?

   ☐ Not offering help or guidance when you need it?

   ☐ Got overly personally involved with you?

   ☐ Not ending treatment when it was not working or was not going anywhere?

   ☐ Therapist seems to be afraid of you when you are dysregulated?

   Others we did not include?

(continued)

3. Of course, it is a dialectic, so it isn't just the therapist having problems. . . .

   Here are some of the TIBs that individuals with problems of emotion regulation, interpersonal sensitivity, or distress tolerance have done that interfered with effective therapy. **Which apply to you?**

   ☐ Nonattendance at individual therapy, groups, doctor's appointments, etc.?

   ☐ Being late to individual therapy, group, doctor's appointments, etc.?

   ☐ Not completing homework or trying treatment recommendations?

   ☐ Noncollaboration in therapy?

       ☐ Passivity or lack of initiative in treatment?

       ☐ Not coming ready with problems to work on?

       ☐ Being so dysregulated the therapist repeatedly has to calm you down?

       ☐ Not reporting what is going on, so you don't have to talk about it?

       ☐ Talking instead of listening in therapy?

       ☐ Pushing the therapist's limits or burning out the therapist?

       ☐ Not doing what your therapist suggests and then complaining that therapy isn't working?

       ☐ Phoning the therapist too much?

       ☐ Making judgments (verbally, with tone, nonverbally) about your therapist?

       ☐ Demanding solutions to problems the therapist cannot solve?

       ☐ Demanding more session time or more than the therapist can deliver?

       ☐ Infringing on the therapist's personal space, etc.?

   ☐ Decreasing your therapist's motivation to treat you?

       ☐ Putting the therapist on the "enemy team" rather than a partner?

       ☐ Assuming your therapist's behavior is occurring because of lack of caring?

       ☐ Impatience and statements the therapist should do better?

       ☐ Criticisms of the therapist as a person, their values, place of work, etc.?

       ☐ Lack of gratitude for the therapist's efforts?

       ☐ Inability to admit progress?

       ☐ Comparison of therapist to other therapists or other people you view as better than the therapist?

       ☐ Overwhelming numbers of gifts, poems, or drawings, etc.?

       ☐ Not taking care of the relationship (e.g., disappearing, not returning calls promptly, making the therapist worry)?

(continued)

153

☐ Talking about suicide without commitment to survive such that the therapist is constantly anxious about your safety or being sued?

☐ Reporting so many nontherapy crises that the treatment focus becomes problem-solving case management issues, rather than therapy.

☐ Showing up very dysregulated—in session or in the waiting room?

☐ Not getting along with clinician's staff or colleagues?

☐ Angry, attacking, or confrontational with lots of judgments?

Others we did not include?

Week 2 Assignment: Therapy-Interfering Behaviors

1. Think through your past treatment experiences and add more to items 1, 2, and 3 on the previous pages.

   a. Interview your therapist(s) (and, optionally, others in your life) to discuss this issue and add additional TIBs of yourself or your therapist(s) on previous pages.

   b. Generate (on your own or with your therapist) a list of the top 10 TIBs *of yourself* that are continuing today, and that you and your therapist will work to change in DBT Next Steps.

1.

2.

3.

4.

5.

6.

7.

8.

9.

10.

(If you come up with fewer than 10 TIBs, be sure to check in with your individual and group therapists for other ideas. If you still have less than 10, congratulations! This, then, is an area of strength for you.)

Week 3: Your Future and Therapy

So . . . with these therapy-interfering behaviors in mind, it is important to think through your choices when DBT Next Steps is completed.

No mental health treatment	DBT Next Steps goal: You are your own therapist for dysregulation and out-of-control behaviors, but might see a therapist for a specific issue on a short-term or periodic basis.
Mental health treatment for a specific problem	
Long-term mental health treatment to remain stable	Very risky: Means relying more on therapy and increasing the chances you will stay entrenched in treatment and potentially end up sliding backward to pre-DBT behaviors or stagnating as you lean more on treatment than on yourself. (Can even be true of DBT if you don't have a predetermined duration of treatment.)

If you attend psychosocial treatment (i.e., not just medications), consider your options:

Another DBT provider	Would allow easy transition and same language; may be expensive. (*Note to the Wise:* Some DBT therapists are scared of client suicidal or high-risk behaviors more than others.)
Individual or group psychotherapist—top person	Getting the best help available; likely to be expensive if they don't take insurance; difficult to get in/easy to get fired; be careful they are not reinforcing ineffective behavior (you are seeing them for their area of expertise so that doesn't make them a DBT/dysregulated behavior expert).
Individual or group psychotherapist—without recommendation	If you are getting better, great. If you aren't, hard to know if it is you or them; likely to be less expensive than the previous options; be careful you are not reinforcing each other's ineffective behavior.
Long-term mental health program	Less likely to include individual therapy; if part of a publicly funded community mental health program, therapists often hired for social work skills more than therapy training. Publicly funded programs in the United States are generally designed to take care of you and protect your rights . . . not designed to get you well enough to leave treatment. (For example, there are frequently state regulations to be sure your rights are protected, but <u>not</u> regulations to be sure that you are given the correct treatment, enough treatment, or evidence-based treatment.) Often, you will only get weekly treatment if you are "sick enough," and if you stabilize,

(continued)

frequent visits will stop. (Does this worry you? It should.) Given this, there is a very high likelihood that treatment will reinforce ineffective behavior and not reinforce self-sufficiency.

You may not be eligible for long-term mental health care if you are working enough to be out of psychiatric disability programs. Thus, ironically, while long-term mental health programs see themselves as a long-term solution, they can only be a short-term solution for DBT Next Steps graduates who are on their way to living wage employment.

Long-term mental health providers are often wonderful, caring people working under extraordinarily difficult circumstances—low pay, high turnover, big caseloads, tons of paperwork. You have to decide if that help is worth the risk of getting lost in the overload.

However, this may be the only good option to obtain psychiatric services, if you are on medication and can't find a private provider or your primary care doctor is unwilling to prescribe your psychiatric medications.

Consider the websites and resources provided by your therapists for finding and evaluating treatment options.

Being the Best Client You Can Be to Get the Best Care

What do the best therapists expect from their patients (and will avoid taking you or fire you for not doing)?

- Show up every week or call to cancel at least 24 hours before the session. (If you cancel in less than 24 hours or are a no-show, pay full price for that session, as insurance will not cover a cancellation.)
- Pay for each session on time and do not continue therapy if you cannot do so.
- Sit quietly and respectfully in the waiting area.
- If you make a mistake, you do not avoid it. Apologize and repair.
- Have a specific issue that you want to work on (not a general "fix me" attitude).
- Allow the therapist to set the agenda (if that's their approach).
- Be a thoughtful consumer and clear on your goals. Talk to the therapist if your goals aren't being met. Listen to their perspective, but don't stay if treatment is not working (and then blame them).
- Be prepared with how you can handle a crisis without needing immediate contact with the therapist. Most therapists do not have 24/7 availability and expect to be called in a crisis at most once or twice during the entire course of therapy. If they think you need more than that, they may not take you on.
- Be prepared to work on what you agreed to work on in the last session.
- Only go off topic for real crisis (not what you can manage but feels like a crisis) and rarely (i.e., less than every 3 months).
- Don't allow yourself to avoid treatment or therapy recommendations and be vigilant to see avoidance coming and talk about it.
- Be regulated and able to focus.
- Have new ideas at the ready, but don't make them more (or less) important than what the therapist has to say.
- Be genuine—if you are trying to look like you have more skills than you do, they feel you are wasting their time (and you probably are). (This is a dialectic for the need to stay regulated, focused, and nonavoidant.)
- Don't act sicker than you are in order to get the therapist to do more, to have more sympathy, or to back off. They will probably do it a few times and then show you the door . . . permanently (e.g., "I'm not sure I'm the right therapist for you. Have you considered community mental health?").
- Be nondefensive when issues in the therapy relationship are addressed by the therapist. (Most therapists consider this completely appropriate to and part of the therapeutic process and are thrown when the client shuts down or won't listen to feedback.)
- If you don't agree with what the therapist is saying, don't challenge them right away. Ask thoughtful, nonjudgmental assessment questions to be sure you understand. Validate. You may want to think about what they've said for a week and discuss it in the next session. (Use DEAR MAN and GIVE as well as FAST.)

**Remember, challenging your beliefs, highlighting internal conflicts,
and generally confronting your view of the world is a therapist's job!**

Week 3 Assignment: Your Future and Therapy

Think through your plans for after graduation from DBT Next Steps and discuss options with your therapist and prescriber (if you will need medications prescribed after graduation).

1. Do you want to be in any mental health treatment after DBT Next Steps? (You don't have to.)

2. If you are on medications and do not have a primary care provider who is willing to prescribe psychiatric medication, where do you want to seek psychiatric services?

   Discuss this with your current prescriber. (If you can't schedule by next week, do this homework as soon as you can and report that to your co-leader when done.)
   What is the next step toward getting this set up?

   When do you need to get started on this (given your graduation date)?

3. If you want psychosocial treatment, do you want psychotherapy or a long-term mental health program? Why or why not?

   What kind of treatment do you want? If psychotherapy, which type?

   Discuss this with your current therapist. (If you can't discuss by next week, do this homework as soon as you can and show it to your co-leader when done.)
   What is the next step toward getting this set up?

   When do you need to get started on this (given your graduation date)?

Week 4: Practice Making Non-DBT Treatment Work

Let's first consider suicidal behavior and other behaviors that scare therapists.

- Have you ever done things that scared your therapist? If so, how recently?
- What is in your medical record? What would previous therapists say if asked without you being present?

Let's role-play in class: One client will be the client who is having thoughts of suicide but does not want to be hospitalized, and a leader will act like a private therapist who is scared by the patient's suicidal thoughts and wants to hospitalize them (or is otherwise feeling out of their depth working with this client).

What strategies did you observe the client using that (1) did not hide what is true, but (2) reassured the therapist, and (3) helped the therapist feel confident the client could cope *without* being referred to the ER or hospital?

What other skills or strategies can the client use? Best strategy: Demonstrate coping—quote examples of skills you can use until the therapist tells you to stop.

Try the role play again.

(continued)

Now, let's consider the TIBs you identified week 2 of this module.

Let's role-play again: One client will be the client trying not to do this behavior but instead be what a top therapist expects, and another client or the leader will act like a private therapist being themself.

What strategies did you observe the client using? What else could they try here?

Try the role play again.

Week 4 Assignment:
Practice Making Non-DBT Treatment Work

Two separate times, role-play effective therapy interpersonal skills in difficult situations. If you have a history of suicide risk, be sure one role play is about suicide prevention. Choose other therapy-interfering situations from your list on week 2 (p. 155). You can role-play with any therapist on the DBT team—try your therapist, your backup, your psychiatrist, or DEAR MAN another clinician.

Describe the first situation you role-played:

Who role-played with you?

Your observations on how well you demonstrated synthesis of the dialectic of both (1) remaining in control of your life and (2) appearing open to feedback and suggestions from the "therapist."

Your role-play partner's observations on how well you demonstrated synthesis of the dialectic of both (1) remaining in control of your life and (2) appearing open to feedback and suggestions from the "therapist."

Describe the second situation you role-played:

Who role-played with you?

Your observations on how well you demonstrated a synthesis of the dialectic of both (1) remaining in control of your life and (2) appearing open to feedback and suggestions from the "therapist."

Your role-play partner's observations on how well you demonstrated a synthesis of the dialectic of both (1) remaining in control of your life and (2) appearing open to feedback and suggestions from the "therapist."

Applications of Mindfulness

Week	Date	Topic	Assignments (due the following week)
1		Mindfulness Practice and Mindfulness to Control Attention	1. Daily mindfulness practice (try different exercises). 2. Mindfulness to control attention assignment.
2		Opening and Refocusing the Mind	1. Daily mindfulness practice (try different exercises). 2. Full participation in the moment—dive into what you are doing.
3		Using the Mindfulness Skills for Anxiety	1. Daily mindfulness practice (stay with one exercise every day). 2. Practice mindfulness for current anxiety.
4		Mindfulness as a Doorway Opening to Skillful Behavior	1. Daily mindfulness practice (stay with one exercise every day). 2. Practice opening to acceptance and to what your emotion has to give you.

Week 1: Daily Mindfulness Practice and Mindfulness to Control Attention

Daily Mindfulness Practice

As part of DBT Next Steps, we want you to experiment with daily mindfulness practice.

Many people around the world have experienced benefit from daily mindfulness.

- It shapes your experience of being mindful and shapes your relationship to mindfulness in a new way.
- Daily mindfulness practice leads to more mindfulness throughout the day.

It is less important how long you practice than that you find a way to make it happen <u>every day</u>.

Practicing mindfulness each day will require planning ahead, problem solving, and (probably) coping ahead.

- Do not assume this will be easy, as most people who meditate or do other daily practice can tell you.
- Assume it will be a challenge, and put time and effort into solving it.

We recommend you consider all the effective strategies that you have learned through Check-In and use them (see the list of Effective Strategies in the Overview, if you can't remember them).

Likely barriers to daily mindfulness practice:

How will you get yourself to practice <u>every day</u>?

During weeks 1 and 2, feel free to try different mindfulness practice to see what works for you. Weeks 3 and 4, pick one mindfulness practice and stay with it for the full 2 weeks.

Mindfulness to Control Attention

How do you know if you are ruminating or worrying?

- If you have been thinking about an issue for more than a couple of minutes and are no closer to solving associated problems/addressing it, then you are ruminating or worrying.
- You are burdened with judgments and describe errors.
- Your thoughts go in a loop—you are going over the same territory repeatedly, obsessing on details.
- It's like being in a hamster wheel—working hard and going nowhere.

Consequences of Rumination and Worry

- Doesn't result in a useful outcome (a.k.a. not effective).
- Causes misery.
- Functions to avoid other forms of pain:
  - Unfamiliar pain
  - Unpredictable pain
  - Pain associated with bad outcomes in the past
- Blocks effective actions:
  - Actions to solve the problem
  - Actions to feel better about the problem
  - Actions to improve acceptance and tolerance of the problem
  - Actions that could lead to more positive events later

Solution: Mindfulness

- Mindfulness is incompatible with rumination and worry.
- Worry time is not rumination or worry (it may look similar, but functions differently).
- Mindfulness is hard to learn, but leads to long-term relief from misery.

(continued)

"Three Mindfulness Strategies"
to Get Away from Rumination and Worry

1. *Mindfulness Exercise* (e.g., observe your breath, imagine spiral stairs)

2. *One-Mindful Action* (i.e., bring your attention to and fully participate in what is effective in the moment)

3. *Mindful Assessment* (i.e., consider the topic of your rumination or worry using Observe and Describe skills nonjudgmentally, one-mindfully, and effectively)

Pick a Mindfulness Strategy you will try this week and decide how you will do it:

Week 1 Assignment: Mindfulness to Control Attention

1. Practice Daily Mindfulness as described on p. 165.

   Describe what you observed about doing it and about getting yourself to do it:

2. Identify at least three contexts in which you ruminate or obsess (e.g., locations, circumstances):

   a.

   b.

   c.

3. What are several topics or subjects about which you tend to ruminate or obsess?

   a.

   b.

   c.

4. Pick one of the Mindfulness Strategies to respond to rumination or worry, and make a cue to remind yourself of it.

   Mindfulness Strategy: _____

   Specifically, I will:

   Pick a cue to check and see if I'm ruminating/obsessing: _____
   (e.g., phone ringing, phone alarm, stoplight, different jewelry, string on finger)

5. Each day, practice that mindful response to rumination or worry *at least three times.*

   Describe what you observed:

Week 2: Opening and Refocusing the Mind

Opening the Mind

Become mindful of everything in the moment, opening yourself to what you have been ignoring or mindless of:

- Pain focuses the mind so it is understandable that you will focus on things related to the pain.
- Fear focuses the mind so it is understandable that you will focus on what scares you.
- There are, however, many other aspects of the situation.

Example: If you don't have much money, then other people get to eat what they want, but you have to eat what you can afford. It takes effort to focus on gratitude.

In-Class Exercise

Remember last night, about an hour before you went to bed; reconstruct that time in your mind. Practice Opening Your Mind. Remember where you were, what you were doing, who and what was there, what you saw, heard, smelled, touched, tasted, etc. Describe as many aspects of the situation as you can—positive and negative, concrete things, body sensations, thoughts, actions.

Of all these things, what were the five you were most conscious of at the time? Where had your mind focused?

(continued)

Refocusing the Mind

Control your attention so that you refocus on the parts of the situation that are most effective.

In times of distress, we tend to narrow our focus on what is wrong. In one audio clip (at https://plumvillage.org/library/clips/enjoy-being), Thích Nhat Hanh offers guidance on how to refocus your attention on the enjoyable aspects of the moment that might be overlooked. This is a shift away from "what's wrong" to "what might be pleasant to observe around me."

The idea here is that there are so many elements in the external world around us, and our internal elements, the feelings, perceptions, and consciousness in our bodies, that are wholesome, uplifting, and healing. Focusing on the negative elements surrounding us can be confining and prolong our misery.

Opening and refocusing the mind mean opening up to the healing elements in your environment and repositioning your mind there again and again. Hanh and Dalai Lama (1992) offer the example of our breathing as a simple way to shift awareness to something pleasant that is with us every moment we are alive. However, many people appreciate the fullness of breathing only when they have asthma or are congested. The idea here is that we don't need to wait until it is adversely affected to fully appreciate our lungs filling with air and emptying out.

Elements like our breath, the clouds above us, the eyes of a friend or someone we care about—all are around us. Each second we are alive is a second to fully absorb these elements. Wherever we are, regardless of the moment we are in, we all have the capacity to enjoy the sunshine, the presence of being in the company of others, the wonder of our breathing. These elements are with us; we simply need to open to and refocus on them. We don't have to travel anywhere, or change up our lives to draw from these elements. Each moment is an opportunity to soak them up (Hanh & Dalai Lama, 1992).

If you made a mindful, Wise Mind choice, what five things would you have placed your attention on? Be careful not to self-invalidate. Allow yourself to nonjudgmentally consider what would have been most effective in Wise Mind.

If you tried to refocus on the Wise Mind things above, which are the "sticky" things your mind would keep getting attached to?

Remember, you can use the Mindfulness Strategies from week 1 to get unstuck.

Week 2 Assignment: Opening and Refocusing the Mind

1. Practice Daily Mindfulness. Change the practice or duration, as needed.

Describe what you observed about doing it and getting yourself to do the practice:

2. One time during the week, practice this exercise on your own.

In a problematic situation, Open Your Mind. Consider where you are, what you are doing, who and what is there, what you see, hear, smell, touch, taste, etc. Describe as many aspects of the situation as you can—positive and negative, concrete things, body sensations, thoughts, actions.

Of all these things, what are the five your mind is focusing most on?

If you make a mindful choice, on what five things will you Refocus Your Mind?

(continued)

Week 2 Assignment: Opening and Refocusing the Mind *(page 2 of 2)*

Which "sticky" ineffective things is your mind staying focused on?

3. One time during the week, consciously embrace what is most important and valuable in the moment you are in.

- Bring every ounce of attention to throwing yourself into and participating in the most important parts of that precise moment, and get everything valuable out of it that you can.
- Accept what is reality in this moment and work from there.
- This exercise is less about Reasonable Mind than exercise 1 above. Don't think; Open Your Mind and Refocus Your Mind, and just experience both.
- Follow Wise Mind wherever it leads you and don't look back.

<u>Afterward,</u> describe:

Situation:

What did you put your attention into?

What was that like? How was it the same or different from your typical experience?

Week 3: Using the Mindfulness Skills for Anxiety

Let's talk about the Mindfulness of Current Emotion skill as it relates to anxiety. How does Mindfulness of Current Emotion work? How do you use the skill with anxiety?

What is the point? How could this help with anxiety?

Research shows that the best treatment for anxiety is Mindfulness of Current Emotion, which most therapies call "exposure" to anxiety. What is it?

The goal of "exposure" is "corrective information." What is that?

(continued)

There are two types of exposure: *"in vivo"* (DBT calls this "Opposite Action") and "imaginal" (DBT calls this "Mindfulness of Current Emotion"). Let's talk about the differences.

What makes imaginal exposure or Mindfulness of Current Emotion for anxiety work well?

How can it go wrong?

Thus, the goal for Mindfulness of Current Emotion for anxiety is that you come to experience anxiety as a wave that comes and goes without causing you injury beyond the anxiety itself. *The outcome of practice is to change your relationship to the experience of anxiety, rather than change the anxiety itself—to one of acceptance rather than suffering.* So, Mindfulness of Current Emotion has value even if it doesn't work as exposure (i.e., if your anxiety doesn't lessen or stop occurring). Exposure is just one purpose.

Week 3 Assignment: Using the Mindfulness Skills for Anxiety

1. Practice Daily Mindfulness. Choose one practice and use it each day for the next 2 weeks. Notice any urges to change practices, but don't make a change.

   Describe what you observed about staying with a single mindfulness practice:

2. Follow the steps below to practice Mindfulness of Current Anxiety:

   a. Have a plan. (This can be discussed with your therapist.)

      • Figure out how you will be mindful of the emotion. Will you practice awareness of body sensations while sitting quietly or walking, practice observing the emotion while continuing to do effective actions, describe in writing to keep yourself focused? Essentially, how will you be mindful of your anxiety?

      • How long do you plan to practice? A few seconds, until the wave passes, 30 seconds, until subjective units of distress (a.k.a. SUDS) go down, 20 minutes, an hour, etc. (Need to end based on when you've decided, not because you can't tolerate it any longer.)

      • Do you need an exit strategy if you become dissociated, psychotic, or otherwise lose control? For example, TIP plus a distracter such as a therapy appointment you have to leave for, scheduled phone call, favorite TV show, another distraction. If so, plan your strategy ahead of time and describe it here.

   b. Start being mindful of your anxiety:

      • "Surf the wave" of your anxiety.

      • Focus on body sensations—attend to the quality of the body sensations and location in your body, noticing changes in intensity or location.

(continued)

- Let go of your expectations and activate curiosity.

- When your mind wanders, smile or half-smile, then bring your mind back.

- Practice loving your anxiety.

- Remember the two "poles" you can hang onto: (i) Remember you have (and will again) felt differently and (ii) remember that you do not have to act on your anxiety (e.g., by avoiding, escaping, switching to anger, blocking).

- Observe any distractions, avoidance behaviors, or thoughts pulling you from one-mindfully participating with your anxiety. Gently return to task.

- Observe any judgmental thoughts or judgmental tones if they arise. Gently return to task.

- After the time you decided on in your plan, step away from the exercise and let it go/shake it off/use exit strategy.

3. Afterward, describe your experience in a few words:
   - General observations:

   - Describe any distractions, avoidance behaviors, or thoughts that took you away from one-mindfully participating with your anxiety:

   - Describe any judgmental thoughts or judgmental tones if they arose during or after the exercise:

Week 4: Mindfulness as a Doorway
Opening to Skillful Behavior

These exercises are alternatives to distress tolerance and white-knuckling your way through a painful or anxious moment.

- This is an acceptance versus change strategy.
- If you are doing this to change your emotions, then you are not doing the right exercise (if they do change, this is a side effect—not the purpose of what you are trying to do).

These exercises are 2–3 minutes long (once you've learned them).

Opening to Acceptance

Opening to Acceptance is useful:
- When willfulness is on board, if you find yourself fighting the emotion.
- To help you be less afraid of your emotions.
- To stick around with your emotions long enough to learn something.
- To stop fighting or suppressing your emotions, so they will stop fighting back.
- To disconnect from the superhighway of thoughts and rumination.

Steps:
1. Pause what you are doing or thinking.
2. Identify the emotion or sensation or experience.
3. Locate it in your body sensations.
4. Move into a body posture of acceptance.
    - For example, focus on your breath, willing hands, half-smile.
5. Find acceptance and willingness.
    - For example, repeat to yourself, "I don't like it, I can't change it, I accept it."

(continued)

Opening to What Your Emotion Has to Give You

Opening to What Your Emotion Has to Give You is helpful:

- To assist you in making friends with your emotions.
- To learn to love your emotions as you do other people, things, and experiences that are important to you (i.e., they don't always make you happy, but they are valuable and overall bring joy or comfort).
- To activate curiosity and change your perspective to one that allows you to benefit or learn from the experience, not just survive it.

Steps:

1. Stop and create a moment to be fully present.
2. Identify the emotion or sensation or experience.
3. Locate it in your body sensations.
4. Move into a body posture of acceptance.
   - For example, focus on your breath, willing hands, half-smile.
5. *If needed*, find acceptance and willingness that your pain or emotion is present.
   - For example, repeat to yourself, "I don't like it, I can't change it, I accept it."
6. Remind yourself that emotions are always valid and this emotion is valid.
   - Know that something triggered this experience.
   - Remember the function of emotions—to motivate, communicate to others, and communicate to yourself.
   - Consider how everything is and everything is caused.
7. Witness your emotion with care.
   - Breathe into your emotion not to change it, but to soothe it, to be present for it, to bring the cool stream of your breath to a hurting body part.
   - Hold it like a delicate flower or a butterfly—hold it steady, protecting it without crushing it.

Week 4 Assignment:
Mindfulness as a Doorway Opening to Skillful Behavior

Practice Daily Mindfulness. Stay with the practice and duration you chose last week. Notice any urges to change practices, but don't make a change.

Describe what you observed about doing it and getting yourself to do it:

Identify two to five situations where your emotions, your fear of your emotions, or your attempts to suppress your emotions limit you or lead you to be ineffective:

1.

2.

3.

4.

5.

(continued)

For one situation that occurs this week, practice **Opening to Acceptance:**

Situation: _____

Go through the steps:

1. Pause what you are doing or thinking.
2. Identify the emotion or sensation or experience.
3. Locate it in your body sensations.
4. Move into a body posture of acceptance.
   - For example, focus on your breath, willing hands, half-smile.
5. Find acceptance and willingness.
   - For example, repeat to yourself, "I don't like it, I can't change it, I accept it."

Observations of process and results:

(continued)

For a different situation that occurs this week, practice **Opening to What Your Emotion Has to Give You:**

Situation: _____

Go through the steps:

1. Stop and create a moment to be fully present.
2. Identify the emotion or sensation or experience.
3. Locate it in your body sensations.
4. Move into a body posture of acceptance.
   - For example, focus on your breath, willing hands, half-smile.
5. *If needed*, find acceptance and willingness that your pain or emotion is present.
   - For example, repeat to yourself, "I don't like it, I can't change it, I accept it."
6. Remind yourself that emotions are always valid and this emotion is valid.
   - Know that something triggered this experience.
   - Remember the function of emotions—to motivate, communicate to others, and communicate to yourself.
   - Consider how everything is and everything is caused.
7. Witness your emotion with care.
   - Breathe into your emotion not to change it, but to soothe it, to be present for it, to bring the cool stream of your breath to a hurting body part.
   - Hold it like a delicate flower or a butterfly—hold it steady, protecting it without crushing it.

Observations of process and results:

Appendices

Name:		

Recovery Goal(s):								
Day of the Week							
Date							

*Mark intensity of experience from 0 to 5.

0 = Didn't happen
1 = Kind of noticed the feeling or urge
2 = Noticed the feeling or urge
3 = Medium feeling or urge
4 = Strong feeling or urge
5 = Very intense feeling or urge
  †List what was done/used, and the number of times in the notes for session below.

‡Rate the skills used from 0 to 7.

0 = Not thought about or used
1 = Thought about, not used, didn't want to
2 = Thought about, not used, wanted to
3 = Tried, but couldn't use them
4 = Tried, could do them, but they did't help
5 = Tried, could use them, helped
6 = Didn't try, used them, didn't help
7 = Didn't try, used them, helped

URGES/OBSER	Suicidal ideation	0–5*						
	Urge to self-harm	0–5*						
	Urge to use	0–5*						
		0–5*						
		0–5*						
ACTIONS†	Self-harm	Y/N						
	Used	Y/N						
		#						
		Y/N						
		Y/N						
EMOTIONS	LOVE	0–5*						
	JOY	0–5*						
	ANGER	0–5*						
	SADNESS	0–5*						
	FEAR	0–5*						
	SHAME	0–5*						
OVERALL SKILL RATING		0–7‡						

Check the boxes below for each day you worked on each skill.

Mindfulness	Wise Mind							
	Observe (just notice)							
	Describe (put words on, just the facts)							
	Participate (enter into the experience)							
	Nonjudgmental (not good nor bad)							
	One-mindfully (only the present moment)							
	Effectiveness (focus on what works)							

Agenda Items and Notes for Session

(continued)

									Agenda Items and Notes for Session
Interpersonal Effectiveness	Figure out interpersonal priorities								
	DEAR (Describe, Express, Assert, Reinforce)								
	MAN—Mindful (Broken Record, Ignore Attacks), Appear Confident, Negotiate								
	GIVE (Gentle, Interested, Validate, Easy Manner)								
	FAST (Fair, No-Apologies, Stick to Values, Truthful)								
	Behavior Change Strategies								
	Finding/Getting People to Like You								
Emotion Regulation	Observing and Describing Emotions								
	Opposite Action								
	Check the Facts								
	Problem Solving								
	Accumulate Positives short term								
	Accumulate Positives long term								
	Build Mastery								
	Cope Ahead (plan + mental rehearsal)								
	PLEASE								
	Mindfulness of Current Emotion (a.k.a. Ride the Wave)								
Distress Tolerance	STOP								
	TIPP—Temperature (dive), Intense Exercise, Paced Breathing, Paired Muscle Relax								
	Pros and Cons								
	Distract (ACCEPTS)								
	Self-Soothe (five senses)								
	IMPROVE								
	Addiction Skills								
	Radical Acceptance/Turning the Mind								
	Willingness/Half-Smile/Willing Hands								
	Mindfulness of Current Thoughts								

NUMBER DAYS COMPLETED DIARY CARD: _____

DBT Weekly Record of Getting Active

Day	Date	Activity scheduling	What I did	Number of Getting Active hours		
				Paid work	Other career activities	Other Scheduled, Structured, Social Activities
Thursday	/					
Friday	/					
Saturday	/					
Sunday	/					
Monday	/					
Tuesday	/					
Wednesday	/					
			Total Hours:			

Getting Active: Includes any activities you and your therapist agree on to expand your engagement in work, hobbies, and leisure, and should generally be activities that are <u>scheduled</u>, <u>structured</u>, <u>social</u>, and <u>out of your home</u>. We particularly want you to break out paid work and other activities to support a career.

Program Requirements: From 4 to 8 months in DBT, maintain at least 10 hrs/wk of Getting Active. From 8 to 12 months in DBT, maintain at least 20 hrs/wk of Getting Active. (*Note:* We ask you to track paid work and other Career Activities as Getting Active because they aid recovery, but they are not required in DBT.)

Name: _____ **Date:** _____ **Number days completed:** _____

Day of the Week							
URGES								
Suicidal ideation							
Self-harm							
ACTIONS								
Self-harm							
EMOTIONS Love							
Joy							
Anger							
Sadness							
Fear							
Shame							

Primary ambition(s) (including but maybe greater than ambition presented in skills-training group):

Agenda Items and Notes for Session

DBT Next Steps Skills and Strategies to Achieve Your Ambition(s) and Recovery Goals:

Home-work Worked on Check-In Action Step.							
Interacted with DBT Next Steps material.							
Worked on assignments for this week.							
Living Wage Employment and Interpersonal Proficiency On time and stayed full-session at work/school.							
Percentage of day followed schedule/time map.							
Did you stay regulated at work/school today?							
Did you use reducing vulnerability skills today?							
Did you use Wise Mind to balance your priorities with others' demands?							
Did you presume nonjudgmental explanation of others' behavior at work/school today?							
Did you avoid something important today?							
No. of times GIVE with new/important person?							
Describe if/how GIVE was experienced by those with whom you work or attend school:							
Building Community Did you meaningfully reach out today?							
Describe if/how GIVE was experienced by friends, family, or partner:							
Did you spend time with people you like and care about? What did you do?							
Did you effectively attend a social event with GIVE? What did you do?							
Self-sufficient Bills paid up:							
Money paid toward debt:							
Money new debt incurred:							
Money put toward savings:							

From your calendar, please note the following for past week:

Hours worked W2 job: _____

Hours of other paid job: _____

Hours of unpaid job in field: _____

Hours attended school: _____

Hours other scheduled activities: _____

Total hours: _____

No. of applications submitted: _____

No. of interviews: _____

No. of contacts asked about jobs: _____

Total: _____

(continued)

DBT Next Steps Diary Card *(page 2 of 2)*

Emotionally Proficient							
DBT skill of the week:							
Experienced fully a wave of emotion:							
Regulated quickly enough to be fully effective:							

Describe efforts toward deadlines with specifics (e.g., dates, who):

Standard DBT Skills—Check the boxes below for each day you worked on each skill.

	Day of the Week							
	Date							
Mindfulness	Wise Mind							
	Observe (just notice)							
	Describe (put words on)							
	Participate (enter into the experience)							
	Nonjudgmental (not good nor bad)							
	One-mindfully (only the present moment)							
	Effectiveness (focus on what works)							
Interpersonal Effectiveness	Figure out interpersonal priorities							
	DEAR (Describe, Express, Assert, Reinforce)							
	MAN—Mindful (Broken Record, Ignore Attacks), Appear Confident, Negotiate							
	GIVE (Gentle, Interested, Validate, Easy Manner)							
	FAST (Fair, No Apologies, Stick to Values, Truthful)							
	Self-Validation							
	Finding/Getting People to Like You							
Emotion Regulation	Observing and Describing Emotions							
	Opposite Action							
	Check the Facts							
	Problem Solving							
	Accumulate Positives short term							
	Accumulate Positives long term							
	Build Mastery							
	Cope Ahead (plan + mental rehearsal)							
	PLEASE							
	Mindfulness of Current Emotion (a.k.a. Ride the Wave)							
Distress Tolerance	STOP							
	TIPP—Temperature (dive), Intense Exercise, Paced Breathing, PMR							
	Pros and Cons							
	Distract (ACCEPTS)							
	Self-Soothe (five senses)							
	IMPROVE							
	Dialectical Abstinence							
	Radical Acceptance/Turn the Mind							
	Willingness/Half-Smile/Willing Hands							
	Mindfulness of Current Thoughts							

Number Days completed diary card: _____

APPENDIX 3. Overview of the Role of the Life Ambition in DBT Next Steps

DBT Next Steps skills training is focused on your life ambition and weekly targets—what you are doing to move forward, step by step, toward a life worth living. While the life ambition is a key part of skills training, this "working document" is at the core of the entire DBT Next Steps approach as it offers the basis for cultivating a more meaningful and satisfying life.

When new clients begin DBT Next Steps skills training, they are asked to create an ambition that is something they passionately want to achieve as a permanent change in their life—a goal that is not the means to an end but an end in itself. Then each week, the clients, with help from the co-leaders and each other, identify an Action Step toward their ambition and an Employment Step that is behaviorally defined, clear when it is completed, under their control, and at which they have a better than 50% chance of success.

For example, one individual's DBT Next Steps ambition was as follows:

"I want to be a highly respected worker who is a key contributor on my team, has insightful ideas, produces high-quality work and is valued, and who is perceived as such by my coworkers. I want to do work that is challenging enough to be interesting, and when it is so difficult that I want to quit, I stick it out and push through it. I want to be a sufficient adult in terms of house upkeep and paying bills on time. I want a relationship where we work as a team and I behave in a way that reduces conflict with my wife by not reacting with defensiveness and actively behaving in ways that cultivate kindness, teamwork, and respect. I want to be a more patient person so that I have the skills to be a kind and understanding dad in the future. I want to live an active and healthy lifestyle where I feel confident that I can meet any challenge that I pursue, including being able to do one pull-up, and one double under (on demand)."

The ambition doesn't need to be this specific, just clear enough to embody the underlying values, and experienced by the individual with enough passion that they have a general direction to work toward. Being a "working document," the life ambition is completed "in pencil, not pen" and is never "final" in order to allow for changes and shifts in the values you prioritize over time. Other DBT Next Steps ambitions could be "Wake up happy more often than not" or "Be the mom my son needs" when these simpler ambitions are at the heart of a life worth living goal. Longer or shorter, the ambition needs to capture what is truly important, meaningful, and motivating for that person. Action Steps for this individual for the week may be to complete financial aid paperwork for school or do 6 hours of studying for the LSAT, or practice a half-smile at one time each day when irritated and take five deep breaths before responding. One Action and one Employment Step are all that is needed each week, although more are acceptable if they fit the individual's ambitions and available time without resulting in partially versus fully completing the Action Steps for that week.

(continued)

This excerpt is adapted from the following book chapter: Comtois, K. A., Elwood, L., Melman, J. N., & Carmel, A. (2021). DBT–Accepting the Challenges of Employment and Self-sufficiency (DBT-ACES). In L. A. Dimeff, S. Rizvi, & K. Koerner (Eds.), *Dialectical behavior therapy in clinical practice applications across disorders and settings* (2nd ed., pp. 207–232). Guilford Press. Reprinted by permission.

During the Check-In section of each DBT Next Steps skills-training session, every client and the co-leaders remind everyone of their ambition and then report on their progress on their Action Step that week and what they did that was effective and any way they avoided working on it. It's an exercise in Opposite Action and Accumulating Positives Long-Term, and everyone is on equal footing, coleaders and clients alike. Consider sharing your ambition using Opposite Action to shame, adopting an alert body posture, looking up at others, and with a confident tone of voice. We ask everyone in the skills training session to practice interpersonal skills by mindfully noticing what is reinforcing to each specific person and actively working to reinforce each other's hard work. Avoidance is problem-solved, and a new action step is chosen and committed to for the following week.

APPENDIX 4. Community Map Example

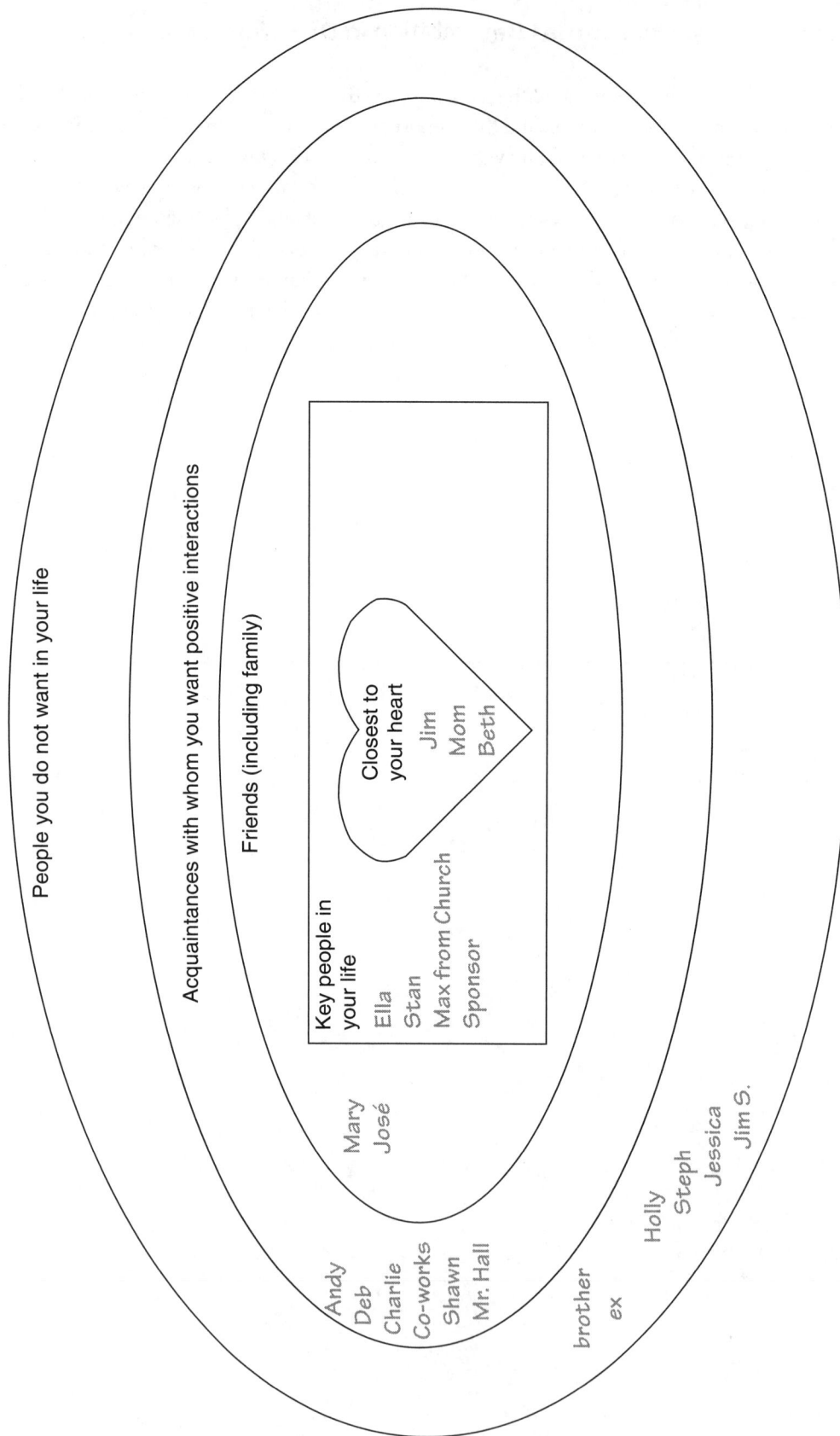

People you do not want in your life

Acquaintances with whom you want positive interactions

Friends (including family)

Key people in
your life

Ella
Stan
Max from Church
Sponsor

Closest to
your heart

Jim
Mom
Beth

Mary
José

Andy
Deb
Charlie
Co-works
Shawn
Mr. Hall

brother
ex
Holly
Steph
Jessica
Jim S.

APPENDIX 5. Ideal Time Map Example

	3/21 THURSDAY	3/22 FRIDAY	3/23 SATURDAY	3/24 SUNDAY	3/25 MONDAY	3/26 TUESDAY	3/27 WEDNESDAY
8:00 A.M.	Read	sleep	Sleep	Sleep	Work (8–2)	Work (8–3)	Bath
8:30 A.M.							Mud mask/nails
9:00 A.M.	Crafts						Work (9–4)
9:30 A.M.		Bath					
10:00 A.M.		Yoga					
10:30 A.M.	Walk the dog						
11:00 A.M.	Nap	Internet	Internet	Internet			
11:30 A.M.		Lunch	Walk the dog	Workout			
12:00 P.M.	Lunch	Meditate	Lunch	Lunch	Lunch	Lunch	Lunch
12:30 P.M.	Check email		Bath	Bath			
1:00 P.M.		Clean	Commute	Cooking			
1:30 P.M.		Break	Dog park	Walk the dog			
2:00 P.M.	Commute			Internet			
2:30 P.M.	Dr appointment	Workout		Time with W			
3:00 P.M.	Commute			Yoga	Meditate		
3:30 P.M.	Email	Walk to cafe	commute		Nap		

(continued)

From *DBT Next Steps Skills Handouts: Building a Life Worth Living*, by Katherine Anne Comtois, Adam Carmel, and Marsha M. Linehan. Copyright © 2025 The Guilford Press. Permission to photocopy this material or download it from the epdf is granted to purchasers of this book for personal use or use with clients; see copyright page for details.

Ideal Time Map Example *(page 2 of 2)*

	3/21 THURSDAY	3/22 FRIDAY	3/23 SATURDAY	3/24 SUNDAY	3/25 MONDAY	3/26 TUESDAY	3/27 WEDNESDAY
4:00 P.M.	Commute	Walk to cafe	Chores	Dinner		Meditate	
4:30 P.M.	Dinner	Walk to cafe	Cooking	Commute	Commute	Workout	Meditate
5:00 P.M.	Food Bank volunteer	Yoga	Commute	Online games	Physical Therapy		Check email
5:30 P.M.			Friends			Chores	Friends
6:00 P.M.		Cook			Dinner at café	Cooking	
6:30 P.M.		Family time				Dinner	
7:00 P.M.					TV with W		
7:30 P.M.		Walk the dog				Meditate	
8:00 P.M.							Chores
8:30 P.M.		Clean				Internet	Cooking
9:00 P.M.						Time with W	Walk the dog
9:30 P.M.	Commute		Getting ready for bed				Yoga
10:00 P.M.	Family time	Time with W	Reading	Chores	Meditate	Write	Time with W
10:30 P.M.	Workout		Getting ready for bed	Getting ready for bed	Yoga		Sleep
11:00 P.M.	Sleep	Sleep	Sleep	Sleep	Sleep	Sleep	
11:30 P.M.							
12:00 P.M.							

References

Barlow, D. H., & Craske, M. G. (2007). *Mastery of your anxiety and panic workbook* (4th ed.). Oxford University Press.

Comtois, K. A., Elwood, L., Melman, J. N., & Carmel, A. (2021). DBT–Accepting the Challenges of Employment and Self-sufficiency (DBT-ACES). In L. A. Dimeff, S. Rizvi, & K. Koerner (Eds.), *Dialectical behavior therapy in clinical practice: Applications across disorders and settings* (2nd ed., pp. 207–232). Guilford Press.

Hanh, T. N., & Dalai Lama H. H. (1992). *Peace is every step: The path of mindfulness in everyday life* (A. Kotler, Ed.). Bantam Books.

Linehan, M. M. (2015). *DBT skills training handouts and worksheets* (2nd ed.). Guilford Press.

Morgenstern, J. (2004). *Time management from the inside out: The foolproof system for taking control of your schedule—and your life* (2nd ed.). Henry Holt/Owl Books.

Pryor, K. (2018) *Don't shoot the dog: The new art of teaching and training.* Ringpress.

Schmidt, J., Lu, T., Boyle, T., & Vedantam, S. (2018, June). *When everything clicks: The power of judgment-free learning.* [Podcast] www.npr.org/2018/06/04/616127481/when-everything-clicks-the-power-of-judgment-free-learning

Index